The Psychology
of Childbirth

The Psychology of Childbirth

AN INTRODUCTION FOR MOTHERS AND MIDWIVES

Joyce Prince
BA BSc PhD SRN SCM

Formerly Principal Lecturer in Psychology, West London Institute of Higher Education
Formerly Honorary Lecturer in Psychology, Institute of Obstetrics and Gynaecology, University of London

Margaret E. Adams
SRN SCM DN (Lond) MTD

Senior Midwife Teacher, Queen Charlotte's Hospital for Women
Examiner to the English National Board for Nursing, Midwifery and Health Visiting

Foreword by
Anne Bent MBE SRN SCM MTD
Lately Professional Officer — Midwifery, United Kingdom Central Council for Nursing, Midwifery and Health Visiting
Lately Director of Education, The Royal College of Midwives

SECOND EDITION

CHURCHILL LIVINGSTONE
EDINBURGH LONDON MELBOURNE AND NEW YORK 1987

CHURCHILL LIVINGSTONE
Medical Division of Longman Group Limited

Distributed in the United States of America by Churchill Livingstone Inc., 1560 Broadway, New York, N.Y. 10036, and by associated companies, branches and representatives throughout the world.

© Longman Group Limited 1987

First edition 1978
Second edition 1987

ISBN 0-443-03388-9

British Library Cataloguing in Publication Data
Prince, Joyce
    The psychology of childbirth: an introduction for mothers and midwives.
    — 2nd ed.
    1. Pregnancy — Psychological aspects
    2. Childbirth — Psychological aspects
    I. Title II. Adams, Margaret E.
    III. Prince, Joyce. Minds, mothers and midwives
    618.2'001'9   RG560

Library of Congress in Publication Data
Prince, Joyce.
    The psychology of childbirth.
    Rev. ed. of: Minds, mothers, and midwives. 1978.
    Bibliography: p.
    Includes index.
    1. Pregnancy — Psychological aspects. 2. Childbirth —
Psychological aspects. 3. Parent and child. 4. Midwives.
I. Adams, Margaret E. II. Prince, Joyce. Minds,
mothers, and midwives. III. Title.
RG560.P734 1987   612.6'3'019   86–26359

Produced by Longman Singapore
Publishers (Pte) Ltd.
Printed in Singapore

Foreword

One of the most exciting and challenging tasks for any author must surely be to write on a subject for a particular profession when there is no similar existing work. This is exactly what the authors of this book have done for the midwifery profession.

Research in the field of the behavioural sciences related to childbearing and family interactions has continued to develop our knowledge and understanding in this field. The value of this book to the midwifery profession and, because of its uniqueness, to a wider readership cannot be overestimated. For those of us who are in contact with the childbearing woman and her family it is essential that we keep abreast of developments in knowledge in the psychology of childbirth.

Readers will surely be grateful to Joyce Prince and Margaret Adams for their hard work in the preparation of the original text and this revision.

London, 1987   Anne Bent

Preface to the Second Edition

In response to helpful comments and discussion with readers and colleagues much of the material in this second edition has been rearranged to correspond to the chronological stages from pre-pregnancy to the new baby at home.

The House of Commons Social Services Committee in its Session 1979–80 examined perinatal and neonatal mortality (HMSO 1980). The Committee expressed concern, amongst other things, over the dissatisfaction that had been voiced by 'consumers' and the need that was apparent to 'humanise the system'. In accordance with a recommendation of the Committee the Government set up the Maternity Services Advisory Committee. The Reports of this committee have provided authoritative guidelines to good practice. Health authorities and the professions are exhorted to make the best use of skills and resources 'in order to provide a more personal and satisfying service for all concerned' (Chairwoman's Foreword to the First Report). Annual Reports of the Health Service Commissioner (the Ombudsman) regularly contain complaints that stem from a lack of understanding between professional and consumer and a failure to make relevant information available to clients and patients.

The relationship between psychology and the reproductive process is now well recognised and the importance of human relations and emotional factors is endorsed in these national reports. Considerable public debate and research has taken place since the first edition of this book appeared. As well as updating the substance of the original we have included two new sections on preconceptual care (or preconceptional care) and on new techniques in human fertilization. Many attitudes to child bearing and rearing are formed well before pregnancy and may affect its progress. Preconception or pre-pregnancy counselling has developed sporadically in the health service so we have tried to give an overview of issues involved.

The Report of the Committee in Inquiry into Human Fertilization and Embryology (the Warnock Report) was published in 1984. Whether or not legislative action on the recommendations is taken, many of the issues that were examined by the Committee are of importance to midwives.

Human relations in childbirth are widely recognised as being of great importance. The midwife's crucial role in influencing many of those relationships is unlikely to diminish and will increasingly constitute an aspect of professional practice for which the practioner is accountable.

J.E.P   London 1987
M.E.A.

Preface to the First Edition

This book started several years ago when we were planning a short lecture–discussion course of psychology for pupil midwives. Until fairly recently midwife and psychologist have had neither interests nor concepts and language in common, and they have therefore had little occasion for communication with each other. Since the 1960s there have been some remarkable developments in the practice of midwifery and obstetrics. Discoveries about the abilities and perceptions of young babies have coincided with these changes. It is becoming increasingly clear that the areas of interest of the midwife and the psychologist are interlocked. Premature delivery, feeding difficulties, the non-thriving baby and non-accidental injury to infants, to take only a few examples, are recognised as being affected by psychosocial as well as physiological factors.

Psychologists are interested in behaviour and experience while midwives concern themselves mainly with normal (meaning physiologically normal) pregnancy, labour and puerperium. Physical and mental events affect one another intimately.

We have tried in this book to bring together ideas, theories, and empirical data which can help illuminate some of the ways in which psychological factors do affect childbearing.

We have coined a new word. The maternalisatum is our term for the whole continuous period from conception to the end of the puerperium. The terms pregnancy, labour and puerperium direct our attention, to some extent, to the differences between them. By the use of a single term we are emphasising the continuity of development which goes into the satisfactory integration of the new child into the family.

We have spent many hours discussing how to translate technical terms and concepts into unspecialised language, and in learning how to see things from the other person's view point. We hope we have devised a book which will be of interest to all those who are concerned with mothers, fathers and babies. Because of its origins it is of prime interest to midwives, though we hope that health visitors, doctors, social workers, district nurses and parents will also find something of value.

Much of the traditional role of the midwife has been abrogated by technical developments in obstetrics. These very developments have created the need for a deeper understanding of the psychological elements involved in reproduction. It is hoped that this book will not only be informative, but also help the midwife to modify and expand her own professional role, and to find new sources of fulfilment for herself and her patients.

The photographs were taken specially for the book by Margaret Adams. These photographs help to demonstrate a few of the aspects of behaviour which we have discussed in the book. They show a few of the many people whose lives we have been privileged to observe, and sometimes to share, at such an important stage. We are greatly indebted to them.

London, 1978

J.P
M.E.A.

Contents

Introduction

The decline in the birth rate and the effective control over reproduction has greatly increased the interest in, and the value of, each new baby. In the developed countries each child born has a very high likelihood of reaching maturity. It is therefore, of great importance that each one should be given the best possible opportunities for development. Advances in midwifery, obstetrics and pediatrics ensure the survival of many mothers and babies who might previously have perished. The active management of labour, which has been the source of much debate in both medical and public press, has solved some problems at the expense of creating new ones. Some of the new issues to be faced by mothers, and those who care for them, before, during, and after childbirth, are of a psychological nature. One of the effects of the technical advances in obstetrics is increased intervention in the biological process of pregnancy, labour and childbirth. Much of the behaviour which is important in the reproductive process is spontaneous and emotional. Many of the changes from primitive to advanced society have depended upon interference with or control of spontaneity. Interference may however distort or change a smooth sequence of behaviour. The mechanisation of labour, and the fact that most babies are now born in hospital, means that there are many ways in

1

which the whole process of childbirth and hence, the relationship between mother and baby is subject to inter-ference by nurses, doctors, midwives, technicians and machines. Research throws important light on psychological processes at work in the formation of attitudes to conception and pregnancy, and of different cultural ideals of the maternal role. The many factors which influence maternal responsive-ness, and the way in which babies develop emotionally, intel-lectually and socially, are relevant to both parents and also those with a professional interest in maternity and child health.

The first chapter reviews some of the changes of attitudes to mothers and babies and the social events which have brought these changes about. How mother and baby get on during their early days together is also discussed, as this is the time when a midwife's care or advice may profoundly influ-ence the course of events.

The course and outcome of pregnancy are much influenced by general health and lifestyle. Effort is now being put into educating both potential parents to 'get fit for pregnancy'. The second chapter highlights some of the issues that are emerging.

Public concern about the possible consequences of man's ability to isolate and control genetic material and repro-duction of the human species led to the appointment of the Committee of Inquiry into Human Fertilization and Embryology. Those aspects of the Report of that Committee that are directly relevant to midwives are discussed in Chapter 3.

Chapters 4, 5 and 6 are concerned with events which primarily affect the mother. Pregnancy is often a time during which preparatory changes are made, both in the personality of the mother and in family structure and arrangements. Pain is often not openly discussed at antenatal classes and we have discussed the need for more information on this subject.

Contraception, amniocentesis, genetic counselling, are relatively recent intrusions in the human reproductive pattern, and views about them become entangled with deeply entrenched attitudes and motivations. Similar difficulties are likely to be encountered in the antenatal period over issues about the termination or maintenance of the pregnancy. Wherever the opportunity for choice is introduced, responsibility is also invoked. This implies taking credit for a commendable outcome and being guilty about an undesirable one. Women have become more conscious of their own role in society, at work, and in families in relation to their husbands and children. The creating of a new baby means also the making of a new role for both parents. The role change is usually more acutely experienced by the mother than the father and some discussion on this is to be found in Chapter 4. The unsupported or unmarried mother often requires special consideration. A number of research reports show the considerable disadvantage to which the children of lone parents are exposed (Ferri 1976, Crellin et al 1971, Report of the Committee on One-Parent Families 1974 The Finer Report). The Finer Report estimated that one-parent families form about a tenth of all families with children and that over one million children are involved. The Finer Report was concerned with families in which the father was the lone parent as well as those parented by mothers alone. Parents may be on their own for a number of reasons. This report does bring home the frequency of the occurrence. The earlier that help is made available the more benefit is likely to accrue to mother and baby. The chapter on labour discusses some of the changes that have taken place in this event in recent years and some possible consequences.

One of the first questions usually asked about the new baby is whether it is a boy or girl. The sixth chapter discusses some of the differences between boy and girl babies, and how the child's sex affects behaviour towards him or her.

Feeding probably occupies more time, energy and thought than any other single activity for several months at the beginning of life, and certainly in the first two weeks. The chapter on feeding discusses the association of feeding with cultural attitudes and with some aspects of the baby's development.

There is always much discussion as to whether a baby can see, hear, think, remember and learn. Since the 1960s there have been a number of ingenious experiments and careful observations which throw new light on these traditional questions. These, as well as some of the many speculations that remain, are discussed in Chapter 9.

The discussion of neonatal abilities leads on to a chapter on physical and psychological development. It is important to try to tease out those factors in very early life which are transitory, and those which may have longer term consequences. It is also important to consider any possibility for reversing the effects of events which may have deleterious long-term consequences. Chapter 11 on the handicapped child looks at some of the evidence available on this question. The birth of a less-than-whole child usually engenders intense emotions in the parents, and often in the professional workers involved as well.

One of the most upsetting events for families and professional workers is infant death. Mothers who have lost a baby often find they are bereft, not only of their child, but of help and support of those around them. Some of the problems involved in communicating about anxiety, depression and grief, are discussed.

In Chapter 13 some factors which are likely to affect the family as a functioning social unit are considered. The paternal role and that of any other children have to be worked out. It is important that a family should have access to as many facilities appropriate for developments as is possible. There are, therefore, some practical guides about facilities that may be available and specialist organisations which deal with particular problems, as well as an introduction to some of the more complex factors involved in the network of relationships in a family.

REFERENCES

Crellin, E., Pringle, M., West, P. (1971) *Born Illegitimate*. Slough: Bureau Books, NFER Publishing Co.
Ferri, E. (1976) *Growing Up in a One-parent Family*. Slough: NFER Publishing Co.
Report of the Committee on One-parent Families (The Finer Report) (1974) Department of Health and Social Security, London: HMSO.

1

Recent changes affecting midwifery

BIRTH AND MORTALITY RATES

Attitudes to babies, child bearing and birth vary considerably from culture to culture, and such attitudes also change over time in any one society. In this country changes, first in the infant mortality rate and then in the birth rate, have had a marked impact on attitudes to child bearing. Two and a half centuries ago the Queen of England, Queen Anne, presumably with access to the best medical advice available at the time, had 14 children, none of whom survived infancy. There is no reason to suppose that this state of reproductive wastage was exceptional, as will be obvious to any casual visitor to a well established Churchyard. The second half of the 20th century in the Western world is very different from any previous period in history in which to have a baby.

In recent years there have been changes in the law relating to abortion, the advent of a nearly foolproof contraceptive pill, the practice of controlled labour, the Sex Discrimination Act, and an increasing number of employed women. Changed attitudes have helped to bring these events about, but the events themselves presage further changes of attitude to mothers, babies and families. A high birth rate, high infant mortality and Sarah Gamp all belong together in a society where many individuals had little opportunity to exert influence or control over their lives or their reproduction. The establishment of midwifery as a highly skilled profession, reflects the social changes which resulted in a fall both of the birth and infant mortality rates. *Laissez-faire* attitudes to birth and babies changed to those of care and concern. It was not until 1902 that the first antenatal bed (one only) was endowed in Edinburgh. The midwife changed in function from the person being 'with the wife' at childbirth, to a person properly educated and trained to understand the requirements for a healthy pregnancy, labour and puerperium. In this role she has been expected to be competent in detecting, and as far as possible preventing, anomalies and abnormalities, to take advantage of medical progress and to help the mother adapt to and manage her new baby.

CHANGES IN OBSTETRIC PRACTICE

Until the late 1960s childbirth was considered a normal process. Improvements in morbidity and mortality of mother and child were sought through improved antenatal care with attention to diet, exercise, early detection of abnormality and so on. Obstetric intervention was considered only exceptionally. Since the late 1960s obstetric practice in the control of labour with induction, acceleration, mechanical monitoring and a readier resort to instrumental delivery has meant widespread changes in the care of women in labour and throughout pregnancy and the puerperium. The question put by Sir John Stallworthy (Professor Emeritus of Obstetrics and Gynaecology at Oxford) to the Twentieth British Congress of Obstetrics and Gynaecology in 1974 has still had no decisive answer. He said that 'it is not yet known whether "office hour obstetrics" will increase the mental, emotional and physical trauma to women . . . or whether it may actually increase hazards to infants by increasing the number of premature babies separated from their mothers in intensive care nurseries'. Widespread concern has been expressed both by members of the professions involved and by the public.

Against the background of these technological changes the midwife's role is changing, and is likely to continue to do so, though not necessarily in the same direction as over the last decade. Home deliveries started to decline following the influential Peel Report in 1970. In this report the risks attached to home and hospital deliveries were compared, to the detriment of the former although this interpretation of the data has been questioned by Tew (1981). A survey by R. G. Law (1967) showed that with grand multiparae the neonatal mortality rate was unexpectedly higher in hospital deliveries. Huntingford (an obstetrician) has been critical that 'new techniques introduced on the basis of reasonable hypotheses were not weighed in the balance. The hypotheses were accepted as proven and new techniques introduced en masse without any attempt to show whether or not they had been proven' (1984). As controlled labour necessitates hospital delivery, the autonomous role of the midwife has largely given place to that of the hospital based midwife, who is one of a team of highly trained technical experts. Both the community midwife and her hospital counterpart, however, try to maintain their continuity of care (though with increasing difficulty), and as such may emerge as the people to whom a woman may turn for advice and interpretation of complex information. In some hospitals, for examples, women are given a choice as to whether they shall have an epidural analgesic or not. How should they come to a wise decision? It is not only a choice of reducing pain for themselves, but of how the baby is likely to be affected, and how the labour is likely to be concluded. (The incidence of instrumental delivery rises with the administration of epidural analgesia.)

Despite changes in obstetric practice, in the midwife's role and in social attitudes, the midwife's traditional interest in ensuring the health of the mother and baby and helping them to get on happily together, remain. The House of Commons Social Services Committee on Perinatal and Neonatal mortality (1980) recommended that 'steps are taken to make better use of the skills of midwife in maternity care – particularly in the antenatal clinic and the labour ward, where they should be given greater responsibility for the care of women with uncomplicated pregnancies' (Vol 1 para 225). If this is to happen administrative action, political will and a restoration of midwives' confidence in their own skills will be essential.

In the past it has been the concern of obstetricians and midwives to help mothers to have physically healthy babies. The perinatal mortality rate (PMR) that is, stillbirths and deaths in the first week of life, has been used as a barometer of success in this endeavour. The downward slope of the curve is cause for reasonable satisfaction (Fig. 1.1), though geographical variations are significant. In 1980, for example, the perinatal mortality rate in Kingston and Richmond in Surrey was 7.6 per thousand: in Walsall it was 19.2 (OPCS Monitor DH3 81/3 6.10.1981). Relatively high rates are also found amongst very young and older mothers (under 16 years and over 34). The social class gradient is also less marked in 1983 than previously (OPCS Monitor DH3 85/2 19.3.1985).

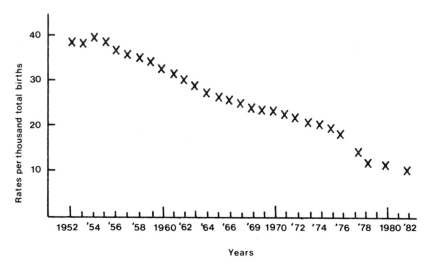

Figure 1.1 Perinatal mortality rate per thousand total births (England and Wales).

CHANGES IN CARE OF THE NEWBORN INFANT

The chances of survival of pre-term, small for dates and sick babies have been improved and their morbidity reduced by the use of special and intensive care. Pregnancy can be very accurately dated by ultrasound. This reduces the risk that babies will be prematurely delivered. In spite, however, of these advances, there does remain a considerable number of babies who spend their first few days in a Special Care Unit.

There are good reasons for believing that mothers who are separated from their babies at the beginning of the child's life, run the risk of difficulty in establishing a good relationship with the infant. With several species of mammal (sheep, goats, monkeys) the mother rejects the infant if the two are separated for the first three days of life. The rejection is the more severe if the mothers are both separated from their infants, *and* placed in a strange environment. If they are together for the first three days and separated subsequently, the mothers accept their babies on reunion. It is a common practice in sheep farming for the shepherd to 'graft' an orphan lamb on to a ewe who has lost her baby by putting the dead lamb's skin over the orphan. A study by Kennel et al (1974) in America shows that human mothers who have their babies with them all the time in the post-partum period, pay more attention to them, fondle and play with them more than mothers whose babies were cared for in accordance with the usual hospital routine, that is, where they spend a proportion of the day in a separate nursery. The difference between the two groups of mothers and babies was still apparent when the children were a year old. Human mothers rarely refuse contact with their babies, though they may express unease about the relationship by saying, 'I can't really take to him', 'What an ugly little thing' or something similar.

There are a number of reasons why mothers may not feel particularly attached to their babies. Whatever the reason may be, it cannot fail to be a source of concern to the midwife. Babies are now highly valued as families are generally carefully planned. There is an accumulation of evidence that the baby who fails to elicit a mothering response, may be at risk in regard to his emotional, social and intellectual development and possibly his physical well-being. There is a higher incidence of non-accidental injury to babies who have been cared for during their early days in Special Care Units. Mothers who came to trial for neglect, cruelty or the killing of their young children, sometimes say that they never had much feeling for the victim, although other children in the family may be satisfactorily cared for. The occasional failure of the mothering response is nothing new. The tradition of the *changeling* child stems from the experience that mother and child seemed not to belong together in the normal way. Throughout history societies have tacitly approved a variety of methods of disposing of unwanted and uncared for babies, from exposure to feeding them ground glass or gin.

The changed attitudes to babies and young children make our response to such events one of very great concern, and make the midwife's role in helping the mother who may be at risk, a crucial one. She is in a central position from which to observe how the infant's behaviour affects the mother, how the mother's behaviour affects the child, and she must also be aware of how her own attitudes may affect them both. For example, in helping a new mother with breast feeding the midwife may be able to teach patience by example, as well as providing practical guidance.

PSYCHOLOGY OF THE NEWBORN

A normal newborn baby probably has much more individuality and more skills than has often been recognised. It is now clear that the newborn infant is not clay to be moulded by his caretakers. He interacts with others and can initiate some sequences of behaviour. Feeding and sleeping problems do not necessarily stem from parental 'mishandling'. Some babies are more irritable than others – they may need less sleep, be more inclined to cry and be generally more difficult to manage. Careful observation and analysis may be necessary if the midwife is to give helpful advice.

At birth it is the usual practice in this country for a midwife or doctor to grade the baby on a number of characteristics to produce a composite Apgar score. Heart rate, respiration, muscle tone, reflex responsiveness and skin colour are each rated on a three point scale (0, 1 or 2) one minute and five minutes after birth. The maximum score is 10 but a score of 8 or over is considered to indicate a good condition. The Apgar score was originally devised for an assessment of asphyxia, so it could be treated more promptly. It has also proved useful in studies of the development of behaviour.

Very low Apgar scores have been found to be related to mental retardation as well as physical handicaps, and intelligence test scores at four years have been found to be related to these Apgar scores. What is perhaps more surprising, is that babies with scores of 7–9, which are considered reasonably normal, do less well than babies with perfect scores, at the age of 3, 9 and 13 months on a test of attentiveness. The children with Apgar scores of 10 concentrated longer and better on pictures they were given to look at. The ability to concentrate plays a very important part in learning and in intellectual development, and its study is important is showing how fairly small differences in condition at birth can affect the individual's development, at any rate within the first year of life (Lewis et al 1967).

In 1973 a Neonatal Behavioural Assessment Scale was published in this country. The author, T. T. Berry Brazelton, an American paediatrician at Harvard Medical School, says in his introduction 'The Neonatal Behavioural Assessment Scale allows for an assessment of the infant's capabilities along dimensions that we think are relevant to his developing social relationships'. It is plain that some babies within a day or two of birth are quite active in initiating and sustaining some kind of social behaviour. This is done by subtle *signals* such as head turning, eye movements and hand movements. The observant and responsive mother reacts to these signals without being entirely aware of doing so, and thus the foundations for communication are laid, upon which a relationship of understanding can be built (Fig. 1.2). Much of the early behaviour of this bond between mother and baby happens too fleetingly and subtly for a human observer to be aware of it. Slowed videotape recording make this awareness possible (Richards 1971). From such recordings it is clear that some mothers can be too active and they then interrupt the baby's sequence of signalling behaviour. In the way that some people who talk rather a lot do not seem to be able to listen to what another person is saying, so some mothers seem to push their side of the communication without giving the baby the opportunity to play his part. This event does seem to be experienced as frustrating for both mother and child.

From studies of the behaviour of mothers with their new

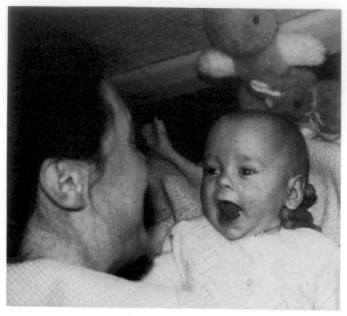

Figure 1.2 Initial stages of communication are made by mother and child responding to subtle signals.

babies it is apparent that features of the infant can affect this behaviour. Perhaps the most obvious thing is his state of alertness. It is certainly not the case that babies are either asleep or in need of food, as has been thought. Brazelton, in his Neonatal Behavioural Assessment Scale mentioned on page 11 proposes distinguishable states which are:

Deep sleep
Light sleep
Drowsy or semi-dozing
Alert, but with minimum motor activity
Eyes open with considerable motor activity
Crying

Anyone having the care of new babies for prolonged periods will be well aware that there are considerable differences between one baby and the next, both in how much time he spends in the various states, and how they are distributed over the 24 hours. The amount of time babies spend asleep has probably been overestimated. In one study the amount of time over 24 hours in the alert but quiet state varied from 4 per cent to 37 per cent of the total time. Perhaps the states which concern mothers and midwives most, are sleeping and crying. Night waking is accepted in the first week or so of life, but it is generally believed that the baby should settle to the normal diurnal cycle sooner or later. If night waking extends beyond about three months the assumption is often that the baby is being mishandled. An enquiry by Richards (1975) into the sleeping habits of babies revealed two important features. One is that sleep problems are quite common, and the second is that the tendency to wake is an individual characteristic of the child which persists during the first year of life and often longer.

In the neonatal period, amounts of sleeping and crying are important and so is the time at which these activities occur. Two babies may cry for the same length of time during 24 hours. The effect this has on their mother will depend on the time at which it occurs. In Richards' study mentioned above, the babies who throughout their first year of life were troubled by night waking, had, as neonates, cried more and had been more irritable and fussy. These mothers had had significantly longer labours, and the babies were slower to cry and establish regular breathing at birth. This points to a fairly persistent individual characteristic of the child. From a practical point of view, advice to parents with a night waking child, may have to take into account the possibility that the problem is to be lived with rather than solved. This, of course, is a difficulty which extends far beyond the neonatal period, but may become apparent in the early days. If, as is suggested by evidence of recent studies, night waking and crying is a pattern of behaviour often resistant to alteration, perhaps mothers can be helped to plan their lives around that fact, rather than being allowed to feel guilty by the suggestion that they are mishandling their babies. Suckling occurring during the night triggers the production of more prolactin than during the day (Glasier et al 1984). Night feeds therefore form an important stimulus to the establishment of plentiful lactation. Practical guidance on such a matter is more likely to be sought from the health visitor or general practitioner than from the midwife. A friend of one of the writers, who had dizygotic twins, one of whom was a night waker for over fifteen months, altered her own sleep pattern to accommodate this fact. Her husband was able to care for the other twin of more regular habit and the elder daughter first thing in the morning until the other two members of the family emerged refreshed! This was a more realistic way of coping, than trying endless manoeuvres to induce the child to change his lifestyle. It is clear that many of them do not. They refuse to accept the long-held adult view that babies are passive and malleable. In some respects they may be susceptible to environmental pressures, but it is important to try to tease out which aspects of their behaviour are fairly individualistic, and which ones are amenable to outside influences.

States of alertness are one of the features of the newborn which depend quite heavily on 'inside' or 'biological' factors, and neither the states nor the timing of them seem to be easy to influence externally. If you watch a baby in deep sleep you will notice that occasionally he seems to *startle* quite spontaneously. Nothing moved his cot, there was no loud noise to disturb him – the disturbance comes from within. Such a startle will sometimes change his sleep from deep to light. The large majority of babies are more responsive to internal than to external changes. Many can sleep though a great deal of noise and movement without stirring, but if they are roused by homeostatic imbalance, they are likely to become more and more alert. In the normal newborn this imbalance is usually very simply accounted for by hunger, for which the baby has a very effective communication system! A small proportion of babies do seem to be relatively sensitive to external stimuli. It is not yet clear whether these early differences have a long term significance.

HABITUATION

One of the important features of the Brazelton test is the assessement it makes of a young baby's ability to ignore outside stimuli. It is important for any living creature to select the signals from the outside world that are significant. Consider yourself walking down the High Street. It is unlikely that you will startle and run from every motor vehicle you hear or see, as you have become entirely accustomed to the noise; so accustomed indeed that you are unlikely even to be aware of it. A novel stimulus may immediately rivet your attention, however, – a pavement musician or the smell of roasting coffee reaches your conscious mind immediately. The process by which we manage to ignore oft-repeated stimuli is called habituation, and the decreasing response is known as response decrement. In the Brazelton test the baby's ability to cut out stimuli successfully is measured in several ways. For example to assess the child's response decrement to light, a torch is shone on the sleeping baby's face. He shows some response by screwing up his face, perhaps moving his head or body. The light is then put off for a few seconds and shone again on his face. This procedure is followed ten times. Babies vary very considerably in their ability to ignore such an irritating disturbance. Some will still be responding to the light after ten trials while others *cut-out* after only two or three. The latter seem to be saying 'There is no harm from that light – I need take no notice'. Those who continue to respond seem to be saying 'I'm still not sure whether this is something I should pay attention to for my own good'. There are high correlations between response decrement to light, sound and pin pricks indicating that the ability depends on some general feature of the nervous system. It seems likely that the baby whose response decrement is fast, will be a relatively calm and placid baby who is fairly easy to manage. This quality will have a considerable bearing on his relationship with his parents. It is important to recognise that babies have very individual ways of responding to stimuli from within and without. Although it may be rather more convenient to live with a placid baby it should not be assumed that there is something wrong with one who does not settle so easily, or who wakes readily.

INFANT FEEDING

Feeding the new baby is of central concern, not only to mother and midwife but certainly to the baby, as he makes clear at fairly regular intervals.

There is a well known correlation between successful breast

feeding and the social class of the mother (Newson & Newson 1963, Sweit et al 1977). Middle class mothers are not only more motivated (in that they plan to breast feed) but they also continue to do so longer. Marketers of infant foods produce very appealing advertisements, as a glance through any woman's magazine will confirm; there is little persuasion on such a scale in favour of breast feeding. There are quite strong psychological pressures which associate breast feeding with immodesty. The breast is a sex symbol and to expose the breast is interpreted as an act of blatant sexual behaviour. If the pressures are to be withstood, the establishment of lactation and feeding have to be associated with satisfaction. The most important satisfaction is a contented baby. In one study done with a group of mothers delivered at home, the mothers were asked to keep a detailed account of what happened during the first 10 days (Richard & Bernal 1972). It was found that breast-feeding mothers fed their babies more frequently (mean number of feeds per 24 hours for breast feeders was 6.6 and for bottle feeders 6.0). The professional advice given to these mothers was that they should feed 4 hourly, missing the very early morning feed. This would have meant 5 feeds per 24 hours. As human milk has a fairly low protein content, it is probable that breast fed babies need feeding rather more frequently. Different species of non-human mammals produce milk that varies over a wide range in its protein and other solid content. Those animals with dilute milk suckle their offspring more or less continuously, while those, like the rabbit, who have very concentrated milk, feed their offspring as infrequently as every 24 hours. Human milk is at the dilute end of the range, and is therefore thought to be more suitable for frequent, if not continuous, feeding. In some cultures babies are carried in such a way that they can suckle at any time. The mother carries the child in a sling in such a manner that her nipple and his mouth are never far apart. In the study already mentioned it was found that crying was more frequent with breast fed babies (Richards & Bernal 1972). Those mothers who continued breast feeding successfully were more likely to respond to the crying by giving another feed, rather than any other kind of intervention. This points to the willingness of successful breast feeding mothers to adapt their routine to the needs of the child, rather than to stick to some preconceived plan. The mothers who, during the antenatal period, had expressed somewhat rigid views about feeding schedules, relinquished attempts at breast feeding fairly readily. The mother's readiness to adapt her routine may be influenced by factors occurring immediately after birth. A study (Sosa et al 1976) in Guatamala shows that when mother and baby are left alone with skin to skin contact for 45 minutes immediately after birth, breast feeding is continued for longer than with mothers who are subject to the normal hospital routine of separation immediately after birth.

Inappropriately made up feeds have been implicated in cot deaths and hypernatraemic dehydration (Taitz & Bayers 1972, Macauley & Watson 1967). There is also evidence that some mothers continually ignore or defy attempts by health visitors to persuade them to make up feeds correctly. This adds to the catalogue of risks to which the bottle fed baby is exposed, and puts a considerable onus on the midwife to help a mother find satisfaction in breast feeding in the first two weeks of the baby's life. Despite the positive views held by the midwife about breast feeding, she may find herself up against some deep laid antagonisms against breast feeding and against accepting babies as they are. She needs a positive attitude to breast feeding herself, and then the time to spend quietly and unhurriedly with the new mother. In hospital the rapid turnover of patients may militate against this. Student midwives and nurses in hospital often lack the experience to help; domiciliary confinements and early transfer home may help the mother to greater success.

Before artificial milk was available babies of the middle and upper classes were farmed out to wet nurses, and breast feeding was associated with a mean and lowly social position. Montaigne, the 16th century French writer, had this to say 'I cannot abide that passion for caressing newborn children which have neither mental activities nor recognisable bodily shape by which to make themselves lovable, and I have never willingly suffered them to be fed in my presence'. The practice of swaddling, common in 17th century England involved binding the infant to a board which was then hung on the wall. Revulsion at many cruel treatments of infants and children is a sensibility recently acquired, and the midwife who does succeed in helping a mother to form a positive approach to breast feeding has to contend with some well established negative attitudes.

MOTHER-INFANT CONTACT

Feeding involves more than the baby's ingestion of food. Giving and accepting food is a symbolic exchange which is central to many social relationships. It is an activity between mother and child which signifies important features of their life together as well as being highly functional. We have already mentioned the evidence showing that the mother who is willing to adapt her routine to the demands of the baby, is the more likely to be sucessful with breast feeding.

It is very difficult, if not impossible to breast feed a baby without being in close physical contact with it! The Harlows' experimental studies with Rhesus monkeys are worth mentioning. They had reared some Rhesus monkey babies with two mother models. One model was made of wire and the other model was covered in terry towelling. Half the monkeys received milk from the wire mother and half from the towelling mother. The two mothers quickly proved to be physiologically equivalent. Monkeys in the two groups drank the same amount of milk and gained weight at the same rate. The two 'mothers' proved, however, to be by no means psychologically equivalent. Records made automatically, showed that both groups of infants spent far more time climbing and clinging to their cloth covered mother than they did to their wire covered mother. They also ran to the cloth covered mother when they were frightened. In fact, they seemed to have grown to love the terry towelling one, who provided comfort but were quite unattached to the wire one even though it provided food. These now famous experiments by the Harlows have some implications for human beings. Contact-comfort, Harlow has argued, is an essential precursor of attachment which forms the basis of a loving relationship (Harlow & Harlow 1966).

The need for attention is perhaps the most compelling human need, which is especially apparent in the very young. Whether close physical contact is the most rewarding attention for *all* human babies is open to question. Some babies are very cuddly and seem to mould themselves to the adult body who holds them. Others, however, rather resist this close contact and hold themselves rigidly. In a study by Schaffer & Emerson (1964) the behaviour of young babies and their mothers was observed carefully. They were all normal caring and responsive mothers and normal full term babies. It was observed that the babies had characteristic ways of responding to close physical contact. Some clearly loved it; others looked rather uncomfortable. Mothers, too, had characteristic ways of dealing with their babies. Some were very much more inclined than others to pick them up, to cuddle them and hold them physically close. These were described as 'handling mothers'. Others were more inclined to speak to, or look at, their baby, to touch him or hold him on their knee in 'non-handling' ways. In Schatter & Emerson's study of 28 babies and their mothers, there were 11 handling mothers, nine with cuddly and two with non-cuddly babies. There were 17 non-handling mothers, ten with cuddly babies and seven with non-cuddlers. The cuddly babies who were mismatched got a lot of cuddling from another member of the family or the mother adapted her own behaviour and gave way to the infant's demand.

The two handling mothers of non-cuddly babies adapted but experienced some embarrassment later on when relatives were faced with the somewhat negative response of an otherwise friendly child when cuddling was attempted. The babies in this study were followed up and non-cuddlers were found to be markedly different in their general behaviour and development from the cuddlers. They reached their milestones of sitting, crawling and standing before cuddlers. The baby who resists the physical constraints of cuddling in the neonatal period may emerge as the individual who, from earliest days, is characterised by vigorous independence. It is important to be clear that an apparent dislike of cuddling does not mean a dislike of attention. The observant and responsive mother can engage in other means of contact. The '*en face*' position, for example, where the mother holds the baby away from her but looks into his face may be a manoeuvre a mother adopts to deal with a non-cuddler (Fig. 1.3). There are 'many factors in the mother's back-

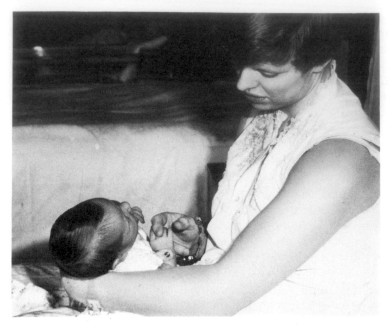

Figure 1.3 Mother making contact with a non-cuddly baby.

ground' that 'can influence how she will relate to her child. . . . Mothers have become rejecting when their babies are unresponsive. . . . But rejection is not a fixed characteristic. Feelings can and do change' (Sluckin et al 1983).

Babies, like other human beings not only like and need attention, but pay attention as well. Periods of alert inactivity, that is, when the infant is fully awake, but quiet, are probably more frequent than is generally supposed. Kleitman (1963) in his evolutionary theory of sleep and wakefulness classified wakefulness into two types: that of necessity and that of choice. Wakefulness of necessity refers to conditions that are initiated by discomfort, such as hunger, cold and bowel discomfort. The periods of wakefulness by choice undoubtedly get longer with maturation, but they are present in normal newborns. A study of Wolff (1965) showed that in the first week of life of ten normal newborn bottle-fed babies, 11 per cent of the time was spent in alert inactivity. This increased to 21 per cent by the fourth week. During periods of alert inactivity the baby's eyes are open, and capable of conjugate eye movements. Some babies become alert and scan the surroundings when they are held to the shoulder for soothing.

Research at Boston University Medical School and St Mary's Hospital, Paddington by Genevieve Carpenter (1970), with babies from one to eight weeks old, shows that from the first days, the newborn plays an active role in selecting the features of its environment to which it will attend. As early as two weeks of age the babies respond differently to the mother's face than to models of a face.

Babies are not infrequently affected by drugs administered to their mothers during labour. The drugs take longer to be excreted by the baby than by the adult, and so the baby may be sedated and unresponsive for a period at the beginning of life. This creates a state of psychological separation between mother and baby which may have some effect on their immediate post-natal relationship. Babies who have been affected by Pethilorfan given to their mothers, have been compared with babies of mothers not given the drug. All babies were normally delivered and healthy. The drug-babies were slower to breathe and cry at birth, the length of their feeds was shorter and their food intake lower. They were sleepy and unresponsive and their mothers tried to arouse them by flicking their feet, or rubbing their legs. On following up these babies clear differences were found at 30 and 60 weeks. The drug babies were found to have fewer social interchanges with their mothers and to be less involved in play activity. They also engaged in more self-stimulating activities, such as thumb sucking, than the non-drug babies though the longer term effects are not known. The state of the infant is one of many factors which can affect the relationship. 'The sex, "look", and temperament of the baby may affect the manner in which the mother initially responds to it,' (Sluckin et al). Positive feelings will develop from rewarding experiences. The midwife may be able to help a new mother (particularly the primipara) to find rewards and to increase appropriate contact between herself and her baby.

The physical care of mother and baby has been vastly improved during this century. A whole and vigorous baby whose mother has difficulty in accepting him is at risk with regard to his long-term development. It is undoubtedly part of the modern midwife's task to ensure that his right to a happy and fulfilling life is not jeopardised by problems created, or difficulties unobserved, in the first weeks of life. There are mothers of babies, indeed families, who need especially sensitive and skilled help to give them a good start. In the multicultural society which we have become, mothers originate from different cultural backgrounds. They come with a variety of attitudes, expectations and values about their family, their marriage and their babies which need to be taken into account. The very young, or the elderly mother, and one who lacks support of a husband or family have special needs. The woman who gives birth to a handicapped, or abnormal child, not only needs help to deal with her own disappointment, but considerable resources to help the baby maximise his capabilities. The mother whose baby dies is a source of very great anxiety; the course of her grief reaction can have radical effects on her family and may affect her attitudes to any subsequent children.

Generally speaking families are very carefully planned and high hopes are invested in each baby that arrives. The decline in the birth rate and in infant mortality has meant an orientation of public interest from child bearing to child rearing. It is now important, as perhaps never before, that every child shall have the best that can possibly be made available to him. This means not only the best in physical standards which we have come almost to take for granted, but the best in emotional satisfactions and opportunities for intellectual and social development. There is now abundant evidence that events before birth, and certainly at and immediately after birth, have an important bearing on these aspects of development. Midwives are especially privileged to be able not only to participate in 'the every day miracle', but also to be in a position to influence the satisfactory formation of the parent/child relationship so essential to the development of the mature adult personality.

REFERENCES

Carpenter, G. G., Tecce, J. J., Stechler, G. & Friedman, J. S. (1970) Differential visual behaviour to human and humanoid faces in early infancy. *Merrill Palmer Quarterly*, **16** pp 91–108.

Glasier, A. S., McNally, A. S. & Howie, P. W. (1984) *Clinical Endocrinology*, 21 pp 109 116.

Harlow, H. F. & Harlow, M. K. (1966) Learning to Love. *American Scientist*, 54 pp 244–272.

Huntingford, P. (1984) The British way of birth. *The Listener*, 9 Aug, vol 112, No 2870.

Kennel, J. H., Jerauld, R., Wolfe, H., Chesler, D., Kreger, N., McAlpine, W., Steffa, M. & Klaus, M. (1974) Maternal behaviour one year after early and extended post partum contact. *Developmental Medicine and Child Neurology*, 16 pp 172–179.

Kleitman, N. (1963) *Sleep and wakefulness*. Chicago: University Press.

Law, R. G. (1967) *Standards of Obstetric Care*. A report on the North West Metropolitan Regional Obstetric Survey, 1962–1964 Edinburgh: F & S Livingstone.

Lewis, M., Bartels, B., Campbell, H., Goldberg, S. (1967) Individual differences in attention. *American Journal of Diseases of Children*, 113 pp 461–465.

Newson, J. & E. (1963) *Infant Care in an Urban Community*. London: Allen & Unwin.

Macaulay, D. & Watson, M. (1967) *Archives of Disease In Childhood*, 42 p 485.

Richards, M. P. M. (1971) Social Interaction in the first weeks of human life. *Psychiatria, Neurologia, Neurochirurgia*, 74 pp 35–42.

Richards, M. P. M. & Bernal, J. F. (1972) An observational study of infant – mother interaction in *Ethological studies of child behaviour*. Ed. Blurton-Jones, N. London: Cambridge University Press.

Richards, M. P. M. (1975) Unpublished lecture delivered at St. Charles Hospital, Ladbroke Grove.

Schaffer, H. R. & Emerson, P. E. (1964) Patterns of response to physical contact in early human development. *Journal of Child Psychology and Psychiatry*, 5 pp 1–13.

Slukin, W., Herbert, M. & Slukin, A. (1983) Maternal bonding, p 84. Oxford: Blackwell.

Sosa, R., Kennell, J. H., Klaus, M. & Urrutia, J. J. (1976) The effect of early mother-infant contact on breast feeding, infection and growth in *Breast Feeding and the Mother*. Symposium 45. London: CIBA Foundation.

Sweit, M. de, Fayers, P. & Cooper, L. (1977) *Lancet*, i 892.

Taitz, L. S. & Bayers, H. D. (1972) *Archives of Disease in Childhood*, 47 p 257.

Tew, M. (1981) Home rule for babies. *Guardian*, 23rd June, p 8.

Wolff, P. H. (1965). The development of attention in young infants. *Annals of the New York Academy of Sciences*, 118 pp 815–830.

Educative function of
  the health professional
Adverse factors

2

Preconceptual care

Antenatal care started with a very modest beginning in Edinburgh early in this century. It was realised that some of the problems apparent at the birth might be ameliorated by care in the antenatal period. Facilities for antenatal care do not usually become available until about the 8th week of pregnancy. During the first four weeks a woman will not know that she is pregnant. There is likely to be a further time lag before the pregnancy can be confirmed. Yet it is in the embryonic stage of development – that is the first eight weeks – that the cell replication and differentiation takes place which lays the foundation for organ development in the fetus.

Nutrient deficiencies, toxic substances and infections are all recognised as being able to influence the developing zygote. A leading article in the British Medical Journal 10 May 1980 pointed out that the infant's 'optimum growth and development are related to the nutritional state of the mother, not only during, but for many years before pregnancy.'

Preconceptual care is therefore a rational extension of antenatal care and health professionals are taking an increasing interest in programmes designed to help improve fitness of both potential parents before the pregnancy begins.

EDUCATIVE FUNCTION OF THE HEALTH PROFESSIONAL

Many matters of general health depend upon self-care and following a lifestyle which promotes well-being: so it is with preconceptual care. A major role for the health professional is therefore an educative one.

Information on the effects of diet, exercise, smoking, alcohol and radiation have had an impact on the general public although changes in behaviour may lag behind the acquisition of knowledge. Many people who appreciate the long-term risks of smoking do not immediately give it up. Most of us learn to like the food we are given as children and adopt it as part of a pattern of life.

Changes in diet entail changes in shopping, cooking, food presentation, and in turn they affect body chemistry. Rituals concerning food are of major cultural importance. There may be some deeply entrenched personal and social habits which cannot be immediately adapted to advice even though its reliability is accepted. All health educators have to grapple with the problem of attitudes, habits and cultural norms which may stand in the way of the long-term goal of improved health.

Preconceptual care focuses several of the general health issues to a specific period in life and for a clearly identifiable purpose. The recipients of advice are likely therefore to be more responsive to information. Many people do make changes in their behaviour when the 'pay-off' is fairly immediate. Some are also willing to make adaptations if there is some prospect that they need not be permanent changes. Prospective parents may be willing to take action for the sake of their baby which would have far less appeal if it were simply for their own long-term benefit. Many women either stop, or reduce their amount of smoking while pregnant. The need to be a good mother is probably more strongly felt, and is certainly more immediate, than the need to look after oneself.

Midwives have been involved in setting up and running preconceptual clinics (Baby Newsline 1985). Concern for the pre-pregnant women extends the midwife's role beyond a formal definition of her work. The field is a relatively new one and there is no national data to provide us with a view about public or professional demand for the service. Chamberlain (1980) in an article on the pre-pregnancy clinic reported on his experience of one such clinic over 18 months. 'By far the largest group of patients were those who had had previous premature labours.' The overt needs of prospective primigravidae are likely to be different from those who have already experienced a pregnancy. The experienced may be motivated to attend in order to avoid a recurrence of a known difficulty. They may require specific advice or possibly treatment, in addition to attention to general health matters which come within the purview of the preconceptual clinic.

ADVERSE FACTORS

Factors which are known to be related to pregnancy outcomes are under- and over-weight of the mother as well as the detailed constituents of her diet. There is evidence that alcohol and smoking may affect both sperm and development of the embryo. Drugs and medicines – including contraceptives (particularly the pill) – must be considered as well as the prospective mother's immunity to rubella. Blood tests may reveal the presence of a problem which may be remediable or of which the couple should be made aware. Information on the occupation of both partners is important. Some jobs in industry, hospitals and laboratories carry particular risks for the developing embryo, for example anaesthetic gases used in the operating theatres. The economic and emotional security of both partners may also affect the progress and outcome of pregnancy. Decisions about breast feeding are often made before pregnancy (see chapter on Feeding) and preconceptual advice may well be beneficial.

It is not our purpose here to suggest specific informational content for a preconceptual programme (see Reference list at end of Chapter). A close relationship between the well-being of one generation and that of the next has been part of general folklore. It is one of the benefits of epidemiological study and microbiological analysis that the mechanisms through which the relationship is mediated are now better understood (Wynn & Wynn 1981). In so far as a midwife has a responsibility for effecting long-term improvements in the health status of the population, she should consider the contribution she can make to the decisions of couples contemplating pregnancy.

Putting theory into practice will necessitate cooperative work with several disciplines – health visitors, occupational health, health education, community medicine and local education personnel. Midwives who work in a family planning clinic are in the best position to advise on the optimum time to have a baby. A health district within West Midland's Regional Health Authority has produced a mobile photographic display and set of slides to publicise the need to 'Get Fit Before Getting Pregnant'. The results of its evaluation are not yet available (Baby Newsline 1985).

This is a developing and important area and there will be much that people can learn from each other's successes, and perhaps even more from their failures. A walk-in clinic has been tried in one area but difficulties in maintaining staff have been considerable. Were details of attempts of all kinds to meet this need to be published, valuable information could be pooled. Research findings on the effects of preconceptual status on the outcome of pregnancy and health of the offspring is the first step. The practical implications of that research and professional responsibility in carrying things forward is the next. The reduction of handicaps in number and degree is the goal.

REFERENCES

Baby Newsline (1985) No 37. *Spring.* Johnson and Johnson.
Chamberlain, G. (1980) The prepregnancy clinic. *British Medical Journal,* 5th July, 29–30.
Leading article (1980) *British Medical Journal,* 10 May.
Wynn, M. & Wynn, A (1981) *The Prevention of Handicap of Early Pregnancy Origin.* Foundation for Education and Research in Childbearing.

FURTHER READING

Know Your Facts No 1 (1983) *Getting Fit For Pregnancy Maternity Alliance.*
Pickard, B. (1983) Nutritional aspects of preconceptional care. *Midwife Health Visitor and Community Nurse,* **19** November.

3

New techniques in human fertilization

The Report of the Committee of Inquiry into Human Fertilization and Embryology under the Chairmanship of Dame Mary Warnock was presented to Parliament in July 1984.

TERMS OF REFERENCE OF WARNOCK COMMITTEE

The Committee had been set up

> To consider recent and potential developments in medicine and science related to human fertilization and embryology; to consider what policies and safeguards should be applied, including consideration of the social, ethical and legal implications of these developments; and to make recommendations. (HMSO Cmnd 9314 p 4)

BACKGROUND TO WARNOCK REPORT

Several years of public anxiety about the implications of advances in the science of embryology, and their application to the alleviation of infertility, came to a head in July 1978 when the first child resulting from in vitro* fertilization was born.

* In Vitro means literally 'in a glass; i.e. the 'test-tube' baby.
In vivo means 'in the body', i.e. the uterus.

The Committee identified two discriminable, though related matters: the possible solutions available to people who are infertile to enable them to create a family; and the scientific development of embryology. Within the first section the implications for the individual and for society of artificial insemination by husband and by donor, ovum donation, embryo donation and surrogate motherhood were considered. Scientific concerns arise from the use of human embryos for research purposes.

MIDWIVES' INVOLVEMENT

We introduce here some of the issues arising from the concerns about infertility, but not those arising from the scientific use of embryos.

In their professional practice midwives have already become involved with the issues that arise from the application of techniques for the treatment of infertility, as an increasing number of babies are being born as a result of successful treatment and some surrogate mothers (though they are likely always to be a very small proportion of the total). They may also be involved in counselling and guidance when potential parents are trying to arrive at a wise decision about possible options for treatment. The issues are somewhat outside the midwife's traditional concerns. Despite this, and notwithstanding the social, moral and legal ambiguities that remain, it seemed to us sensible to include reference to the topic in an attempt to highlight the issues that have a bearing on midwifery.

Infertility may be caused by total or relative failure to produce ova or sperm, by a mechanical defect in the reproductive system of either partner, or by some incompatibility between the male and female reproductive system. Modern techniques enable ova or sperm to be supplied by another person to overcome the first problem. Mechanical defects of the reproductive system can be overcome either by surgery or by using gametes from either the partner's themselves or from some other person(s) and effecting fertilization in vitro and transferring the zygote for implantation to the woman of the partnership or some other woman. The incompatibility between male and female reproductive systems can be overcome by similar methods.

The possibility arises therefore that one or both biological parents (who supplied the genetic material) of the resulting child are different from the social parents (who want him and will look after him).

SIZE OF THE PROBLEM

The extent of involuntary childlessness in our society is not known and one of the Committee's recommendations was that this should be rectified by an appropriate collection of statistics. It was also recommended that each Health Authority should review its facilities for the investigation and treatment of infertility. Dissatisfaction was expressed about the haphazard organisation of services and the often low priority given to problems of infertility. As we write in mid-1986, Government action has not yet been taken on any of the recommendations of the Report and it is therefore the case that the services available lack a coherent structure.

COURSES OF ACTION

Artificial insemination

A couple who wish to embark on treatment of their infertility may, during the course of the necessary investigations and treatment, have to consider the involvement of another person or persons as sperm or ova donor, or as providing a uterus for implantation of the fertilized egg cell. The other person may be one who will donate sperm for artificial insemination into the woman of the partnership. It may be a woman who will donate an ovum for transfer into the uterus of the infertile woman. It may be a man and a woman who donate sperm and ovum which are fertilized outside the body and then transferred to the uterus either of the infertile woman or to another woman who has agreed to carry the child for the period of the pregnancy.

Artifical insemination by the husband (AIH) is technically a simple matter though morally objectionable to some. The

Warnock Committee advocated its use except in the situation where the husband had died leaving frozen semen in a bank. Profound psychological problems to mother and child were thought to be a possibility and should not therefore be risked.

Artificial insemination by donor (AID) can be used where the husband is infertile or where there is a risk of transferring a hereditary disease carried by the man. Despite considerable early disapproval of AID the practice has grown. The legal position Is that neither AIH nor AID is unlawful, though in the case of AID it is the donor who retains the parental rights and duties over any resulting child, not the husband of the child's mother. As the practice will continue to grow the Warnock Committee recommended that it should be properly organised, permitted only by practitioners licensed for the purpose, and that the status of the child and that of the husband of the child's mother should be legitimated.

In vitro fertilization

Techniques for artificial insemination have been available for about 40 years. The extraction of ova, their mixture with semen outside the human body and transfer of the fertilized ovum back to the uterus is a recently developed technique known as in vitro fertilization (IVF). The technical difficulties of transfer to the uterus for implantation are considerable. To maximize the chance of success more than one fertilized ovum is transferred: commonly four. The excess of fertilized ova may increase the risk of multiple birth but more important from an ethical point of view is the issue of what shall happen to those surplus embryos who have been brought into existence but cannot be further sustained.

Ovum donation

An extension of the IVF technique is in egg donation. An ovum can be collected from a fertile woman in the course of some other operation, fertilized and transferred to the uterus of the woman of the infertile couple. Unlike semen, however, ova do not survive freezing. The need for precise timing adds considerably to the difficulties of the technique.

ETHICAL PROBLEMS

1. Identity of biological parent/s

The Warnock Committee considered whether parties to these interactions should be known to one another. They recommended anonymity between the infertile couple and the donor. They did however recommend that the child, on attaining 18 years, should 'have access to basic information about the donor's ethnic origin and genetic health . . .'

2. Surrogacy

The Committee set its face firmly against surrogate motherhood – that is the use of a third party as a carrying mother, as 'the danger of exploitation of one human being by another appears . . . . . . to far outweigh the potential benefits' (para 8.17).

3. Inbreeding

They were also concerned about the possibility of semen from one donor being too widely used. The remote possibility could arise of unwitting incest between children of the same donor. The risks of transmission of inherited disease were also considered and the committee recommended that a limit of 10 children from one donor should be maintained for the present.

STATUTORY CONTROL

The field of reproductive technology is at present in this country formally uncontrolled. There is no licensing authority so practitioners are not required to adhere to any agreed code of practice. The legal status of the parties involved is sometimes ambiguous.

AMBIGUITIES FOR THE CHILDREN

Little, if anything, is known of the children (and their families) whose existence has arisen from the successful application of one or other of the techniques available. Adopted children have often experienced doubt about their own origins and difficulties with their self-concept. Ambiguities of a similar nature seem unavoidable where biological and social parenting are discreet. 'The power which microbiology and biomedicine have given us to regulate and interfere with the reproduction of the species requires, if we wish to retain our humanity, that we re-think what we are about, what we value in each other, children, women and men, and how in the new circumstances we can achieve those values.' (Stacey 1985)

Midwives have a critical role to play in any re-thinking about what is of value and how it might be attained. Scientific discoveries and technological achievements have a neutral value. It is how they are used that invests them with possibilities to advance or retard human happiness and well-being. It is unlikely that the midwife will have had a part to play in decisions about artificial fertilization but she will be required to attend the parents during the process of child-bearing. It is essential that the midwife should consider not only her own moral stance but also that of the parents and support them in the normal non-judgemental professional way unless asked for her opinion.

REFERENCES

Report of the Committee of Inquiry into Human Fertilization and
    Embryology (1984) Cmnd 9314. London: HMSO
Stacey, M (1985) *Journal of Medical Ethics*, 11 No 4 pp 194.

4

Antenatal events

During pregnancy a woman prepares herself for a completely
new role. The first pregnancy means modifying a wife and
worker role, to accommodate to a mother role. Subsequent
pregnancies entail changing from the mother of one child to
becoming the mother of two. Appropriate role behaviour
means living up to expectations and demands of society as
they are manifested through neighbours, relatives, newspaper
and television. There is universal recognition of the mother
role, and little ambiguity about what constitutes proper role
behaviour. A good mother is required to care for her baby,
to feed, clothe and keep him warm. She is expected to
provide opportunities for his physical, intellectual emotional
and social development. Most women become progressively
aware of these requirements which will be made of them
when their baby is born, and put considerable thought and
planning into equipping themselves for their new role.

INFLUENCE OF EARLY EXPERIENCES

Human beings have long, if selective, memories, and there
will be many such memories for the pregnant woman to
revive, stemming from her experiences of her own mother,

and others with whom she has had an important relationship. She is likely to remember consciously or otherwise her own mother; the mother's attitudes to her daughter are likely to become part of her own attitudes to her coming baby. If she had an unsatisfactory relationship with her mother she may hope she will manage things in a better way. If her own early life was contented she is likely to accept the idea that she will get on well with her baby, without much question. Much of the memory of early experience may become distorted with the passage of time but the feelings associated with the memories will nevertheless be real. Recollections of things past are likely to be interwoven with hopes, fantasies and fears about the future.

Harlow's experiments (Harlow & Harlow 1966) with baby rhesus monkeys reared with artificial mothers have been mentioned elsewhere in this book. These monkeys who had grown up without a real mother, and without any experience of another of their own species, were very difficult to mate. The few females who did become pregnant were hopeless mothers. They neglected and ill treated their babies.

In a study done at St. Thomas' Hospital it has been found that women who had been separated from their mothers in the early years, had more difficulty in adjusting to their maternal role, and experienced more problems not only with their babies but with their marriages (Frommer 1973). This study provides support for the idea that some aspects of motherhood are transferred from one generation to the next in quite subtle ways. Some girls not only have a better relationship with their fathers than their mothers; they may also identify more with their fathers. That is, they aspire to being more like their father than their mother. Masculine traits of ambition, assertiveness, activity and self-confidence have become more socially acceptable in women in the past twenty or thirty years. It is believed that the daughter who has identified with her father may find more difficulty in adapting to the pregnant role. She may postpone the starting of a family until later than is usual. Some psychoanalysts (Menninger 1943) claim that psychological masculinity and physiological femininity cannot go together happily. This view does seem to overlook the fact that having and caring for a baby requires not the passivity, submissiveness, and receptivity which are claimed to characterise the typically female personality, but considerable forward planning, energy and vigour. Past experience of intimate relationships affect a woman's feelings about herself, by providing her with models and referants.

Psychological development is a long and continuous process. Early experience is of very great importance, and learning goes on throughout life. Societies vary in their attitudes to pregnancy and motherhood. Some societies for example have a place of very high esteem for the pregnant woman, and delivery is thought of as a joyful event. Infertility is often regarded as a curse, or due to some evil supernatural intervention. There is likely to be an easy acceptance of the pregnant and maternal role in such a culture. In our own society attitudes to pregnancy are not so straightforward. The first pregnancy often means relinquishing a job, and the financial independence that goes with it. Social evaluation of people derives in part from their income, and one of the damaging aspects for anyone who is unemployed is the loss of status suffered. By no means all women do give up work; the point is that it is quite permissible to do so and this affects attitudes to pregnant women.

PREGNANCY AND THE 'SICK ROLE'

Another area of conflict which has emerged in this century is the association of pregnancy with medical care and hence with illness. The first antenatal hospital bed was provided in Edinburgh in 1902 (Donald 1972). From an obstetric point of view, the developments which followed were highly desirable and no-one would want to return to the high maternal and infant mortality rates of the past. The fact that a considerable amount of antenatal care is provided in a hospital setting, however, inadvertently reinforces the view that pregnancy is pathological. Rosengren (1961) found that women who regarded pregnancy as an illness, have significantly longer labours. This can be interpreted as showing that the illness role carries with it expectations of behaviour which the subject endorses. Margaret Mead (1950) in her anthropological studies has found that in some cultures morning sickness is expected for primiparae only, in some it is always expected, and in others it is regarded as abnormal. The numbers of women experiencing morning sickness varies with social expectations. Recent developments in obstetrics can only strengthen the association between pregnancy and illness. Pregnancy is *diagnosed*, there may be some discussion about a *therapeutic* abortion, an amniocentesis to make a *diagnosis* of the condition of the fetus, ultrasound cephalometry which involves some medico-technical procedures, and finally delivery itself has become mystified in medical technology. Pregnancy, which in some societies is seen as the peak of female vigour, health and good fortune, is in the advanced societies a confusion of low status, illness, pleasurable anticipation and fulfilment.

Role conflict often produces a state of inactivity at best, depression at worst. If we occupy two roles at the same time and they make equally strong but different demands, this can result in chronic indecision and inactivity. The person in such a position is often confused not only over what to do, but also unsure whom she is. Some women avoid the role conflict by avoiding pregnancy altogether. Ellen Peck's *The Baby Trap* (1973) is a spirited attack on what has been described as the myth of motherhood. The myth is the idealised family, the carefree mother and the beautiful babies, as presented by the food and clothing manufacturers' advertisements, the women's magazines and some of the material published by the health educators. The reality behind the myth is rather different as we know from discordant families, unhappy distraught mothers and neglected injured children.

CHOICE AND CONFLICT

Another reality is that the improvements in the position of women have in some ways made their lives more difficult. They have more freedom of choice. Any choice point can become a conflict point. Ann Oakley (1975) has shown that in 1971, 60 per cent of women who stopped work did so because of pregnancy, whereas in the 1930s and 40s the usual reason they gave up work was marriage. This means that the first pregnancy is for many women a time of considerable identity crisis. Ann Oakley reports a young pregnant woman as saying 'I can picture myself going out to work but I can't picture myself looking after a baby . . . I'd like the experience of having a baby and then I'd like to give it to someone else to look after and go out to work . . . It's very boring at home. I won't be able to talk to anyone . . . I'm scared of everything.'

Ellen Peck's solution to the identity conflict is to recommend avoidance of the motherhood role altogether. For many women this is not a suitable answer: they really want babies. A few women can perhaps, like Ellen Peck, dichotomise the problem into either motherhood, or social and economic freedom and independence. Many would prefer to work towards a society where bearing and rearing children can be integrated more smoothly into an active social and economic life.

Dana Breen (1975) draws attention to two contrasting assumptions about pregnancy which underlie some particular studies and much of our thinking about the state. These two assumptions she calls the *hurdle* and the *development* assumption. *Hurdle* thinkers consider pregnancy as a period of deviation from normality, with a return to some former state when it is all over. The *hurdle* concept is implicit in such statements as 'All pregnant women are slightly unstable', 'Several researches find pregnancy is associated with an increased neuroticism score'. The suggestion is that when the pregnancy is over stability and a low neuroticism score will reassert themselves.

Development thinkers on the other hand, look at it as a phase of maturation and growth, which results in a new and more elaborate organisation of the personality. Adolescence as a developmental phase has attracted more interest than has pregnancy. There are some parallels. The adolescent has to contend with rapid inner physiological and psychological changes, and at the same time changes in psychological and social demands made of him by others.

It is a period of considerable role conflict – is he an adult or child – dependent or independent? Both the adolescent and those with whom he lives, learns, and works, change their views and behaviour about him from hour to hour. There is abundant evidence of the behavioural consequences of the conflict experienced during adolescence, but the great majority can eventually integrate their inner experience with external demands and opportunities, and emerge as more developed, integrated and competent personalities. In pregnancy too, there are inner physiological and psychological changes, which coincide with changing expectations by others. The role conflict between wife, worker, mother, independent or dependable person, is likely to be experienced as some sort of crisis. A crisis can be seen as the point at which established patterns of functioning are found to be ineffective. Its resolution comes about with the discovery of new effective modes of thinking, feeling and behaving. The identity crisis may begin some time during pregnancy, and continue for a considerable time after the baby is born. Behaviourally we need a single term to cover the four episodes of pregnancy, childbirth, puerperium and early motherhood. For want of an appropriate word let us call the period the *Maternalizatum*. It begins with fertilisation, and is complete when the woman has adjusted the integration of her maternal role with her total personality. This process needs a lot of experience and learning. In less advanced societies where girls and young women take part in the care of other people's babies, much of the necessary experience is acquired before pregnancy. Few girls in our present society have any experience of handling small babies and little time is given to cultivating parenting attitudes in boys and girls at school.

ANTENATAL DEPRESSION

There are a number of studies which show how isolated and depressed women at home with their small children feel. Hannah Gavron's *The Captive Wife* and *Stuck at Home* by Susan Lovegrove are two such examples. It is now emerging that a considerable number of women are depressed in the antenatal period. A Swedish study (Nilsson 1970) found significant psychological disturbance in 25–30 per cent of women attending antenatal clinic. Results are awaited from a similar study now being carried out in the antenatal clinic at University College Hospital, London.

While the problems of the young woman, isolated by her house-keeping and childminding role, have been acknowledged for some time, it has perhaps not been so readily recognised that the dispiriting, debilitating problems, perhaps arising out of role change and personal conflict, are present in a proportion of women antenatally.

Few midwives would feel competent to diagnose psychiatric problems but if these findings are replicated in other antenatal clinics it is plainly of importance that they should be able to do so. We have elsewhere referred to the midwife's role in the continuity of care, and it is in the antenatal clinic that this function should begin, and here that she can start a relationship which can continue until after the baby is born.

THE ANTENATAL CLINIC

Improvements in medical care require increasing specialisation and the effects of this can be experienced by the woman in the antenatal clinic as a series of discreet interests. Her antibodies, weight, baby's head size concern individual people and between them all 'she' is lost. Some women have complained that the only thing that anyone seems the slightest bit concerned about is the baby. One woman said 'As far as they (at an antenatal clinic) are concerned I'm just a vehicle for carrying this baby about – no thoughts, no feelings of my own – nobody asks how I am.' Few sacrifices are made without resentment. When expectant mothers are made to feel that they have some sacrificial duty to their babies they may subsequently be less able to deal with them without hostility. They will have been dutiful but disliked it. To some extent we are all affected by the *we-must-like-babies* folklore. The myth itself often prevents realistic expression of dissatisfaction with the pregnancy. This may be one of the factors underlying depression in the antenatal period. Perhaps midwives should have more training and practice in the management of aggressive and hostile expressions. It is a fairly normal response to feel alarmed if someone speaks destructively or even resentfully of their baby but a midwife is in a very good position to help a woman to recognise her own feelings and perhaps to help her make use of them for her personal development.

A woman in her thirties pregnant for the first time said of herself at the antenatal clinic 'I'm surprised at myself. We've waited such a long time for this baby and now it's coming I'm not so thrilled. Everyone else in the family is very excited and I seem to be dragging my feet over it all.' After a little more discussion the midwife was able to say 'Perhaps you feel as if you are being taken over?' She agreed and they were able to proceed to talk about feelings of resentment at the loss of autonomy.

The Maternity Services Advisory Committee to advise 'on matters relating to the maternity and neonatal services' was set up in 1981 in an effort to further reduce the perinatal mortality rate. The then Minister of Health, Dr Gerard Vaughan, is reported to have said that women were not satisfied with antenatal clinics. They found them badly organised, unfeeling and ineffective. 'We must encourage pregnant women to go to antenatal clinics and make them more welcome' he said. 'Many women go once and never again. Many women who should be screened for possible complications do not attend until late in their pregnancy' (Guardian 1981). Robinson (1983) has shown that midwife and obstetrician replicate each other's work in physical examination in the antenatal clinic, and yet needs of women for advice and support often go unattended.

A proportion of pregnancies end in an abortion. In 1971 for 74 pregnancies that produced a child it is estimated that there were 15 which ended in a spontaneous abortion and 11 which were medically terminated (Lafitte 1972). The miscarriage of a much wanted baby can occasion a marked grief reaction. Several writers have suggested that spontaneous abortion can result from the inability to resolve the inevitable conflict of being pregnant. Jean Hanford (1968) has suggested that there are two stages in resolving this pregnancy conflict. Even when the pregnancy is wanted the emotional stress arising from the adaptations which have to be made, produce a rise in the blood levels of histamine and steroids. As the pregnancy proceeds psychological defence and development take place and the physiological response is lessened. For some women who experience intense conflict, however, the psychological adaptation is insufficient. The irregularity of corticosteroid levels then continue and this can damage the fetus and can lead to spontaneous abortion, prematurity and fetal malfunctioning. This theme of damage being caused to the fetus by emotional stress and psychological conflict has been expanded by Pasamanick in his proposition that there is a continuum of reproductive casualty. We will return to this later in the chapter.

ANTENATAL INVESTIGATIONS

It has been estimated that in 1984 85 per cent of pregnant mothers in England had an ultrasound examination some time during their pregnancies (RCOG 1984). A Medical Research Council (1985) report says the benefits of routine scanning of fetuses outweigh any known risks. The RCOG report recommends that 'mothers should clearly not be persuaded into having the examination against their will and those hospitals which practise routine ultrasound should include a written explanation in their antenatal booklet as to why the procedure is recommended. Scanning personnel should establish that mothers have read and understood the explanation before performing the examination. It is very important that both parents fully understand what investigative procedures of ultrasound and amniocentesis involve. Lay people complain with considerable regularity that medical personnel do not make themselves understood and do not listen, or do not make themselves available, to their patients. (For a more detailed examination of this problem the reader is referred to a collection of papers called *Medical Encounters* edited by Horobin & Davis 1977). Any consent to operation or treatment is intended to be informed consent. Where the question of giving consent arises it is doubly important that the midwife should spend time elucidating the procedure and its purpose and to deal sympathetically with whatever enquiries the patient or her husband may wish to make.

RECOMMENDATION FOR ABORTION

The result of the amniocentesis or ultrasound may lead to the recommendation of an abortion. Nobody has to have an abortion and no doctor, nurse or midwife is compelled to have anything to do with it if she or he has conscientious objections. There are many people who may have moral misgivings without being conscientious objectors. On one hand there is a biologically scientific attitude to the problem which does not acknowledge that any moral issue exists. On the other is the view that the calculated destruction of any form of life is immoral, if not sinful and can never be countenanced. Most people are probably somewhere between the two extreme views and could be persuaded that on some occasions an abortion is absolutely right and on others absolutely wrong.

The pregnant woman is not only the carrier of a fetus. She may be the mother of other children, somebody's wife, a neighbour, a daughter; she is part of a matrix of human relationships of which the fetus will become a part. It is this total web of relationships and the rights, demands, expectations which they involve which often have to be weighed in the balance when therapeutic abortion is being considered.

The majority of recommendations to abortion, and requests of women for it, are carried out. Reaction to abortion varies. A Norwegian study (Kolstad) of 897 women reports that 82.5 per cent were glad without reserve 9.8 per cent were satisfied but doubtful, 3.8 per cent were not happy but realised the abortion had been necessary. 3.7 per cent were repentant. A total of 4.3 per cent had some serious mental disturbance. Similar studies generally show the majority are satisfied but with a very small percentage experiencing some long term mental problem. So far as we are aware no study has yet been done which adequately takes into account the original motivation for the abortion. In view of what has already been said about role conflict and its effect on functioning, abortion even when induced, can be seen as a conflict resolution.

Where amniocentesis or ultrasound have revealed an abnormality, informed counselling will be essential. Some problems are known to be much more likely in families where they have already occurred – for example with *spina bifida*. The risks of recurrence of genetic abnormality can sometimes be mathematically calculated. In the end, however, no parents can be assured that their next pregnancy will be satisfactory, nor can they be certain that it will not be. Nothing is certain; it is the parents who have to weigh the risks of failure against the possibility of success. In order to do this they need the most accurate information that is available and ample opportunity to discuss the pros and cons. A well informed and trusted midwife who knows not only the biological factors involved but something of the social background, the hopes and fears of both parents, can serve as an invaluable guide in the process of arriving at a decision.

EFFECTS OF ANTENATAL EVENTS ON THE FETUS

Obstetricians and midwives, it is often emphasised, deal with two people at a time. While the mother is adjusting to her pregnant role and thinking about her new baby and how she will behave as a mother, the fetus is developing at an extremely rapid rate. Growth is never again so fast. The uterus accords considerable protection from external stimuli to the fetus, but this is to a very large extent offset by its extreme sensitivity. When growth is very rapid stimuli may have a disproportionately powerful effect. It is now well established that a variety of agents which affect the mother also effect the developing fetus. Drugs, smoking, inappropriate diet, radiation, infections, pollutants have all been incriminated in fetal damage. There is also clear evidence that psycho-social factors experienced by the mother affect fetal development.

Studies with animals have the advantage that conditions can be precisely controlled. During the 1930s the injection of certain chemicals and hormones or the deprivation of vitamins to pregnant mammals increased the incidence of various malformations in the offspring. It was suggested that each species or strain had genetic *potentialities* for malformation which are *facilitiated* by exposing the unborn animal to an adverse intrauterine environment. Pregnant animals exposed to anxiety in the form of fear of an electric shock (which is never given) have infants who are timid and disinclined to explore.

Pregnant laboratory mice have been observed to miscarry if the mother perceives the smell of a strange male on the nesting material. These two examples show that fertility can be reduced or offspring impaired by psychological events (that is where the influence is by way of the mother's sensory perceptions).

There is a variety of studies which relate overcrowding in mammals to reproductive difficulty. Animals, however, are not human beings and it would be unwise to assume that the human fetus is exposed to similar risk without further evidence.

There is pronounced association of socio-economic status with the incidence both of obstetric problems (Butler 1969) and with low levels of intelligence and achievement (Vernon 1969). The perinatal mortality survey found that the reading scores of children at seven years of age whose mothers smoked during pregnancy were significantly lower than those who did not.

Closely related to socio-economic status is population density and this is known to be associated with obstetric problems and with child behaviour problems. Many factors are likely to be involved here both pre- and post-natally. Overcrowded rodent mothers however, produce infants with impaired learning ability, increased emotionality and increased timidity (Keeley 1962).

Stott (1963) has shown that infant ill health, malformation, defect of temperament and mental subnormality form a syndrome which is highly related to stress in pregnancy. The stress he has investigated was occasioned by the experience of housing difficulties, marital infidelity during the pregnancy or bereavement. The idea that emotional upheaval for the mother affects fetal development is an old one. It had been abandoned as being unscientific (presumably because the maternal and fetal vascular and nervous systems are quite separate) and has only been reinstated in the fairly recent past.

Newton et al (1979) have shown that stressful psychosocial events during pregnancy may precipitate premature labour. If antenatal care is to have a beneficial effect in reducing the impact of such stressful events it must offer an understanding ear and psychosocial support as well as physical care.

Pasamanick and Knoblock (1966) have proposed that there is a continuum of reproductive casualty. They suggest that an adverse event during the antenatal period may have an effect on the fetus ranging from fetal or neonatal death through a series of sublethal but handicapping conditions, including learning and behaviour problems. It is suggested that a factor which is known to increase the risk of fetal death (for example rhesus incompatibility) is likely in milder forms to produce a handicapping condition. Likewise a number of mildly disadvantaging factors may be cumulative and manifest their effects in physical or psychological abnormality. The continuum can be represented in the following figure (Fig. 4.1).

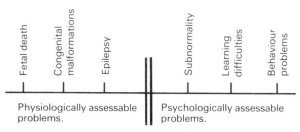

Figure 4.1 Diagrammatic representation of Pasamanick's continuum of reproductive casualty.

Although there is evidence to support the general thesis that a wide range of physical and psychological events impinging on the mother affect the developing fetus and affect it in some graduated way, the details of the continuum have yet to be researched in detail.

In the diagram above it will be seen that conditions to the left of the line are physiologically assessable while those to the right become apparent only through behaviour.

Behaviour is seen to be more sensitive an indicator of prenatal adversity than is physiology. The effects of drugs, prolonged anxiety, infection and so on, on the fetus may be insufficient to affect the infant's morphological structure but may, nevertheless affect neural tissues during their development and hence affect learning ability, responsiveness and long term behaviour.

The idea of a continuum of reproductive casualty is important for the midwife for two major reasons. It suggests that a wide range of physical and psychological events can affect fetal development. It also puts physical and psychological development of the fetus in a coherent and continuous relationship.

ANTENATAL EDUCATION

The 1970s and 80s have seen a great growth of interest in community health and self-help. The DHSS consultative document Prevention and Health: Everybody's Business (1976) summarised much of the thinking on the matter. The midwife in her care of the antenatal mother can play an important part in encouraging community health and self help by including in antenatal classes an education programme.

Antenatal preparation varies from district to district and may be undertaken by a variety of professionals. The Court Report (Report of the Committee on Child Health Services 1976) made a plea for more information to be made available about the function and achievements of parentcraft classes associated with antenatal clinics. Parentcraft, however, is not the only education endeavour undertaken during the antenatal period, and here we summarise, and comment on, some of the factors which are concerned. It would be wrong to suggest that this is an exhaustive summary and equally wrong to suggest that all antenatal clinics follow the same pattern. There is no nationally agreed curriculum; so much depends upon the local interests and enthusiasms.

Most antenatal classes have high informational content. Few women have any detailed knowledge about the growth of the fetus and antenatal education provides a good opportunity to discuss fetal growth, the changes in maternal metabolism and the requirements for the maintenance of optimal health of mother and fetus. In the course of such discussion the value of antenatal visits can be made clear. Later in the pregnancy information about feeding and breast preparation is often included. In view of the findings of Eastham et al (1976) mentioned in Chapter 6 that over half the 200 women in his survey had made up their minds about preferred method of feeding before the pregnancy, the timing of the presentation of this material needs careful consideration. There is a case for thinking that if attitudes to feeding are to be influenced, the earlier breast feeding is discussed the better.

Some preparatory classes include information about the process of labour, and guidance as to what the mother might expect in the way of management during labour, particularly regarding types of pain relief available. In some cases this is combined with a tour of the hospital and labour ward, so that the strange environment is made less threatening when labour does begin.

In addition practical training is often given about relaxation or psychoprophylaxis. The husbands are sometimes included at this stage. Many people take the view that a woman's husband is likely, if she requests his company, to be a good source of moral support during labour. Some are of the opinion that as a joint parent he has a right, if he wishes, to be present at the birth. The current practice in most hospitals seems to be to allow husbands into the labour ward if their wives wish it, and on the understanding that they will leave if requested.

There is the hope, although as yet little evidence to support it, that the parenting role of the father will be encouraged by his being involved as fully as possible during the pregnancy, labour, and delivery. The Court Report (*Fit for the Future –* 1976 p. 115) has this to say: 'A sense of responsibility and partnership is also more likely to be developed if parents are enabled and encouraged to discuss with their advisors the arrangements for the baby's birth'.

Discussion of the sort envisaged here needs to cover not only practical matters but feelings and attitudes of both parents to the coming baby and some consideration of the father's role.

There is probably, in most antenatal preparation classes, an inadequate recognition of the emotional adjustments required of both parents and little discussion on the matter. Referring to fathers one midwife is reported as saying 'They can make a sort of barrier between the midwife and the mother . . . And, of course, they faint.' (*Radio Times*, 19–25 March 1977, p. 68.)

This seems to dismiss fathers as having no place at the birth of their children. A further extract from the Court Report reads 'This report would also like to see a further study of prenatal care with clearer guidance on what advice parents need during the antenatal period and how best to give it' (*Fit for the Future –* 1976 p. 117).

'The once forbidden subject of "pain" must be freely

discussed' (McKenna 1976). There has in the past been some thinking that women suffered pain because they had been led to expect it. The devoted practice of antenatal exercises which it was believed would lead to a painless childbirth often led to bitter disappointment, a rapid crumbling of morale and a fear that the pain signified abnormality during labour. There are so many variables in culture, education and attitudes of an antenatal group that it requires a skilled teacher to respond to all needs.

In a study by Charles et al (1978) there were no differences in obstetric outcome to a group of women who had taken psychoprophylaxis training (as compared with those without training), but they did experience lower levels of pain and multiparae needed less analgesia.

The Court Report is concerned by the possibility of conflict between the hospital and the community professionals giving the classes. Many midwives have not had the opportunity to develop their teaching skills since qualifying, and student midwives often lack details which our sophisticated society demands. Health visitors may have had only twelve weeks obstetric training, so although trained to educate, often lack the wealth of practical experience needed for the session of teaching about labour.

The future course of labour and its outcome are unknown. The majority will have normal deliveries but a small minority will need highly specialised care. All these eventualities cannot easily or beneficially be discussed in the group as a whole. Some information about the range of analgesics, their method of administration, the likely effects on both mother and baby, are sometimes discussed.

In the past decade there have been innumerable books, leaflets, television and radio programmes on aspects of child-bearing. Parents are becoming better informed. The antenatal classes can capitalise on this information but also need to give special consideration to the less well informed mother and father. Patients who have had their babies often display a great fund of goodwill to the hospital staff and to other mothers. Some would undoubtedly be willing to come to antenatal classes to give the consumer's side of the picture.

THE FATHER'S ROLE

The antenatal period is a time of change for all members of the family. The changes in the social role of women have been accompanied by considerable changes in the role of men. Many expect to participate in the care and upbringing of their children. Ours is now a multiracial society, however, and it must be remembered that some immigrants fairly newly arrived in the United Kingdom come from a very different cultural background where the male and female roles follow the traditional pattern of being almost entirely separate. Perhaps nowhere is this separation more clearly marked than in the bearing and caring for babies. Men from traditional societies would probably find a close association with the proceedings of an antenatal clinic embarrassingly novel. Their wives are unlikely to welcome any sudden change in behaviour either.

Nevertheless all couples, immigrant or indigenous will, during the antenatal period undergo some change in their relationship in anticipating the baby's arrival. The first pregnancy means a modification for the husband to a husband-and-father role.

Some men marry in order to be mothered and cared for. The need to share the motherly person they married may not be entirely welcome, nor is adjustment particularly easy. The relationship between sex and parenting drives has not been systematically explored. It is generally assumed that the 'natural' state of affairs is that the sex drive is stronger in men and the parenting drive stronger in women. Masters & Johnson (1966) have produced evidence which calls the former assumption into question. The parenting drive may be largely learned. Women with no experience of babies seem to have little 'natural' gift to guide them. Men often seem quite as strongly motivated to have children as women do. These two elemental forces of the family, sex and parenting, are not always equally valued by both partners. 'I married a lovely, sexy girl – then she turned into someone's mother . . .' reads a comment from a marriage guidance counsellor's client.

The partners in a marriage develop and change and the pregnancy is a period of potentially rapid personality growth for both. It is a fortunate couple who find that the pattern of their expectations, values and fulfilments progresses reciprocally. Biologically the mother experiences greater change and this is mirrored in the expectations that she, her husband and society have of her. An expectant mother publicly proclaims the fact in her changing shape. The expectant father in Victorian tradition was little more than a figure of fun – a superfluous male in female world. One can only speculate rather gloomily on the effects that this derisive attitude has had on the family. Both men and women probably now have greater personal expectations of the marriage relationship than their grandparents did. (For a further exploration of this thesis the reader is recommended to Ronald Fletcher's *The Family.*)

The expectant father role is at present in process of being defined. The trend is certainly towards a much more active involvement of the father with events during the maternalizatum (see p. 39 this chapter).

It is probably true to say that the father role is easily understood in relation to older children. Babies, by tradition are seen as relating primarily to their mother. It has been found, however, that the development of early attachments may be to more than one person and is sometimes primarily made with the father. Schaffer and Emerson (1964) found that over a quarter of 58 babies they studied selected father as the chosen attachment object.

The midwife's activities, advice and guidance during the pregnancy are likely to affect the attitude of both parents to each other to the pregnancy and therefore to the baby when he arrives. This is perhaps a particularly important factor when we consider the father's position. He may, initially, be unsure of what is expected of him. The development of the expectant father role may turn out to be of great importance in the maintenance of family relationships and therefore in providing a suitable environment for the development of the child's full potentialities. If as we think a midwife should take broad consideration of the family happiness and the infant's long term development into her reckoning, appropriate steps to achieve these objectives have to be taken as early as possible.

THE SINGLE MOTHER

The unsupported, unmarried mother usually causes the midwife considerable concern. Unmarried and unsupported are not necessarily the same thing; what matters is whether the mother has a relationship with someone who can make suitable economic provision, help her and generally share the joys and frustrations of caring for the baby. Social security provides for a minimum standard of living so that no woman should be destitute. There is more to life than material survival, however. There is sharing and communication, understanding and learning from a relationship that derives its meaning from the opportunity it gives the participants for personal and social growth.

A woman on her own with a young baby is denied much of this opportunity. To love her baby she needs to experience love herself. Unmarried mothers do not have a monopoly of this deprived emotional life, however. Every marriage does not develop in the way the partners may have originally hoped. They may quarrel, or the marriage can quietly decay for lack of common interests, and an absence of demands and rewards. The pregnant wife of such a marriage may be economically secure but psychologically unsupported. Conversely a woman without a husband may have a good and loving relationship with someone who can provide her with the necessary emotional sustenance. This provision is occasionally made by parents. The risk they run of usurping the maternal role is, however, obvious, particularly if the expectant mother is herself little more than a girl.

So the midwife has a dual concern; one for the material facilities and support that the pregnant woman has available; the other for the affectionate and caring relationships she has. These two factors will enter into consideration if the possibility of abortion is reviewed. Should abortion be unacceptable the question of the baby being adopted may then have to be discussed, although this is now rare.

Abortion or adoption may be a solution in some cases. Despite appearances there are probably few truly accidental pregnancies. Some single women plan their family with as much foresight as a well regulated married couple. For some a pregnancy is disastrous, perhaps affecting educational or career prospects, threatening established relationships and upsetting families. For most unsupported mothers the position is neither a disaster, nor the outcome of careful calculation but somewhere between. The midwife has to keep the welfare of both mother and baby in mind. If the mother wants to keep her baby she will need as much support as she can get and it will be worth discussing with her what resources she has – is the baby's father interested? Or will her own family help her? Young women from some immigrant groups can be rejected by their own people and are in a pathetically isolated situation. There is the young woman who has known little of a caring family life herself, who is highly, but unrealistically motivated to have a baby thinking that he will provide her with the loving and belonging experiences of which life has cheated her. Unfortunately such young women rarely have the resources to enable a baby to learn affection from them. Nor do they realise the demands an infant will make. The risk of mother and child eventually separating to create the same problem in the next generation is quite high.

THE SCHOOLGIRL MOTHER

The problem of schoolgirl mothers has increased in recent years. Disturbed adolescent girls are often shy, timid and inhibited and little complained about because they cause no nuisance. The small proportion who do act out the troubles of disordered and conflict-ridden homes at adolescence often do so by sexual misconduct. This may be promiscuous or through the formation of a strong but quite unsuitable relationship. Their indiscriminate search for the affection which they have not experienced at home can make havoc of their young lives.

The situation in the last decade has been changed by a more general acceptance of pre-marital sexual freedom and a relaxation of restrictions on adolescents both concerning their sexual behaviour and the availability of contraceptives. The age of maturity has also been decreasing for some time. Patterns of adolescent sexual behaviour have probably changed since Schofield's study *The Sexual Behaviour of*

Young People (1964) but this is to some extent a matter of speculation. It is probably the less well organised girl, with personal and family problems, who is the more likely to become pregnant, however, and to present herself as one of the least able to contend with the demands of unsupported motherhood.

During the antenatal period adoption may be the course decided upon. An adoption is usually arranged through an adoption society, a local authority or, until recently, a 'third party' i.e. their own parents or some other individual.

Whether she decides on abortion, adoption or to keep the baby, the unsupported mother, whatever her age or background needs the best facilities that can be made available.

REFERENCES

Breen, D.(1975) *Birth of a First Child*. London: Tavistock Publications Ltd.
Butler, N. (1969) Perinatal Problems. 2nd Report. *Perinatal Mortality Survey*. Edinburgh: Livingstone.
Charles, A. G., Norr, K. L., Block, C. R., Meyering, S. & Meyers, E. (1978) Obsetric and psychologic effect of psychoprophylactic preparataion for childbirth. *American Journal of Obstetrics and Gynaecology*, **131** (1).
Donald, Ian. (1972) *Practical Obstetric Problems*. Edn., p. 3. London: Lloyd Luke Medical Books.
Eastham, E., Smith, D., Poole, D., & Neligan, G., (1976) *British Medical Journal*, **1** pp 305–307.
Fletcher, R. (1966) *The Family & Marriage in Britain*. London: Penguin.
Frommer, E. A. (1973) *British Journal of Psychiatry*, **123** No. 573.
Gavron, H. (1966) *The Captive Wife*, London: Penguin.
Guardian (1981) *New Committee to Fight Baby Deaths*. 17th July.
Hanford, J. (1968) Pregnancy as a state of Conflict. *Psychological Reports*, **22** (3). pp. 1313–1342.
Harlow, H. F. & Harlow, M. K. (1966) Learning to Love. *American Scientist*, **54** pp 244–272.
Horobin, G. & Davis, A. (1977) *Medical Encounters*. London: Croom Helm.
Keeley, K. (1962) Prenatal Experience on Behaviour of offspring of crowded mice. *Science*, **135** p 44.
Kolstad, P. (1957) Therapeutic Abortion. *Acta Obstetrics & Gynaecologica Scandinavia*, **36**. Supplement 6.
Lafitte, F. (1972) *New Society*. **22** No. 532 pp 622–626.
Lovegrove, S. (1976) *Stuck at Home*. London: BBC Publications.
McKenna, J. (1976) Antenatal preparation and epidural anaesthesia. *Midwife, Health Visitor & Community Nurse*, **12** No. 3 pp 78–81.
Masters, W. H. & Johnson, V. E. (1966) *Human Sexual Response*. Boston: Little, Brown.
Mead, M. (1950) *Male & Female*. London: Victor Gollancz.
Menninger, W. C. (1943) The Emotional Factors in pregnancy. *Menninger Clinic Bulletin*, **7** pp 15–24.

Newton, R. W. Webster, P. A. C. Binu, P. S., Naskrey, N. & Phillips,
  A. B. (1979) Psychosocial stress in pregnancy and its relation to the onset
  of premature labour. *British Medical Journal*, 2 pp 411–413.
Nilsson, L. (1970) *Acta Psychiatrica Scandinavica*. Supplement 220.
Oakley, A. (1975) The trap of medicalised motherhood. *New Society*. 34
  No. 689 pp 639–641.
Pasamanick, B. & Knoblock, H. (1966) Retrospective Studies on the
  Epidemiology of Reproductive Casualty. *Merrill Palmer Quarterly*, 12 (1),
  7.
Peck, E. (1973) *The Baby Trap*. London: Heinrich Hanau Publications.
Prevention & Health: Everybody's Business (1976) DHSS. London: HMSO.
Radio Times (1977) pp 19–25th March. London: BBC Publications.
The Report of the Committee on Child Health Services (1976) *Fit for the
  Future*. p 115. London: HMSO.
Rosengren, W. R. (1961) Some social psychological aspects of delivery
  room difficulties. *Journal of Nervous & Mental Diseases*, 132 (6)
  pp 515–521.
Schaffer, H. R. & Emerson, P. E. (1964) The development of Social
  attachments in Infancy. *Monographs of the Society for Research into
  Child Development*, 29 No. 3.
Stott, D. H. (1963) How a Disturbed Pregnancy can Harm the Child. *New
  Scientist*, 320.
Vernon, P. (1969) *Intelligence & Cultural Environment*. London: Methuen.

5

Labour

Many women find the final four or six weeks of pregnancy extremely tedious. Their cumbersome size and shape prevents easy movement and they tire easily. Labour is inevitable and the prospect of its commencement is often welcome, despite apprehensions as to what is in store. Preparatory classes in the antenatal period may have provided some factual information as to how the baby will be born, and what can be expected during the course of labour. No one, however, can know how they will feel about the experience. Even women who have already had a child may find they have quite forgotten the details of the event. Preparation for labour in the antenatal period can involve both expectant parents. Most primigravidae will have very little idea about how the labour is likely to begin, when they should come to the hospital, or summon the midwife, and what is likely to happen after labour has begun. This information about the physical aspects of labour is often reassuring to both parents. Fathers who have been hesitating over whether to accompany their wives during labour can often come to a rational decision about the matter, when they have a clearer picture of what it entails, and what might be required of them. The physical and mechanical aspects of labour are well understood by the midwife. There is yet much to be discovered about the psychology of parturition although no one doubts the important part which psychological factors can play.

It is evident that women from different cultural backgrounds behave differently in labour. They respond to cultural expectations and norms. Some expect the experience to be agonising and behave as if it is so; others that giving birth is part of the annual round occasioning a brief respite in the day's work. There are shouts, groans and grunts, or quiet decorum which are broadly characteristic of the culture. The influence of past experience, of expectation, of ideas about childbirth, and about her own body are all likely to affect the behaviour and experience of a woman during labour. 'So childbirth may be experienced according to the phrasing given it by the culture, as an experience which is dangerous and painful, interesting and engrossing, matter of fact and mildly hazardous, or accompanied by enormous supernatural hazards' (Mead 1950).

FATHERS IN THE LABOUR WARD

In the past few years it has become accepted, in most places, that fathers may if they wish, stay with their wives in the labour ward. The modern management of labour has virtually eliminated prolonged labour which was often distressing to the patient and onlookers, and has been a factor facilitating the involvement of husbands. Many fathers to whom we have spoken are delighted to have taken part in the event and they certainly sound as if their relationships with their children are richer for having seen the very beginning of their independent life. Some systematic study of fathers in the labour ward is necessary in order to assess the importance of various factors. The experience may have a profound effect on their parenting behaviour and therefore on family life in general. A husband can be a great comfort, simply by being present during the labour. A short play called 'That's my Baby' showed the relationship between husband and wife during the antenatal period and during the labour. They had made up their minds before the labour that it was going to be a *natural* one. The husband took on the important role of protecting his wife from the persistent attempts by the obstetrician to administer drugs, send the husband home, and generally interfere to control the course of events. It was an excellent illustration of the fact that, for obstetricians and midwives, the understanding of physical events of childbirth is often far in advance of the understanding of the psychology of parturition. A recent survey published by the Association for the Improvement of Maternity Services (AIMS) has shown that over 80 per cent of women who have experienced both home and hospital confinements preferred to have their babies at home (AIMS 1975). At home the mother is surrounded by people and objects with which she is familiar, and she and the baby are central figures in the family drama. The domiciliary midwife has usually had prolonged contact and establishes a close relationship with the mother and family. Lady Micklethwaite, President of the National Childbirth Trust wrote 'Our experience, in close contact with parents before and after childbirth, has taught us that good emotional support and encouragement during labour can not only reinforce the effect of any drugs that need to be given for pain relief, but can sometimes mean that this kind of medication is unnecessary' (*The Sunday Times* 1974). The favourable rating of home confinements by those women with the necessary experience to make informed comparison, must surely be derived from the value they attribute to intangible factors. They feel happier with people they know on their own territory, where they are understood and where they are in a web of established relationships. The most ardent advocates of home confinements have never claimed the technical equipment is superior to that of hospital. The easy communication and good relations which characterise a contented family is rarely experienced in hospital. These may be important factors which are in need of special attention by the midwife looking after women in labour in hospital.

In general, hospitals have found that inhibitions to a free flow of information, and discussion, have a measurable effect on both staff turnover and the speed of patient recovery (Revans 1964). Learning is essentially a 'feed-back' process, and depends upon seeing the effect of one's own behaviour. Without a flow of information uncertainty increases and with it anxiety. It is the anxiety which affects staff morale and patient recovery. It also increases the subjective assessment of pain.

MOTHER'S SELF-CONCEPT

In midwifery, as in medical practice generally, the patient as a source of ideas and initiative has been underrated. This has led inadvertently to a serious undermining of the positive contribution which a woman feels she can make to labour. Kitzinger (1971) reporting on communications received by the National Childbirth Trust from mothers says 'It is intended that the mother shall feel secure and confident but when she asks a question she may well be told "Leave it all to us, you can trust us to decide what is best for you", or even, "What's it got to do with you? You mind your business and we'll mind ours!"' These responses, and many similar emphasise to an alarming degree the divorce between physiological and psychological understanding. Actually giving birth to the baby becomes somebody else's responsibility. The dilatation of the cervix, position of the fetal head are undoubtedly important concerns. So too, is the significance and meaning a woman is able to attribute to the whole event. Is childbirth simply a matter of the mechanical progress of the baby through the birth canal, or the final exhilarating experience of bringing forth the life which has been nurtured unseen, but felt within, for so many weeks? The significance of that new life for the mother, father, the family can be enhanced by an acknowledgement of the family relationship which have brought it into being, and which will influence its further development. Mothers usually know little of biparietal diameters, and pelvic measurements. What they do know is that they love or hate, are euphoric or depressed, feel the positive motivating force of the contractions or the pain of resisting them. A woman may feel during labour that the baby is, as it has been for the preceding months, an integral part of *her* physically, mentally and spiritually. On the other hand, she may feel it to be a parasite, whose disfiguring dependence is shortly to come to an end. To view the process of labour as simply a mechanical exercise, is to overlook the significance of the feelings of the mother. An exclusive emphasis on the physiology of childbirth can demean the individual mother to a more-or-less efficient reproductive system, and make trivial her important contributions not only to the course of labour, but to events which follow it.

The hurdle concept of pregnancy mentioned in Chapter 4 applies equally to labour. To view it as a temporary aberration from normal, or as a temporary illness, obscures some of the positive developmental processes that are possible. That is not to overlook the abnormal developments which may take place during labour and require urgent intervention. In the last decade techniques which have been found to be effective in the treatment of abnormal obstetric conditions have been increasingly applied to normal ones. The modern management of labour entails the application of three techniques. They are, induction of labour, the administration of oxytocic drugs and epidural analgesia. (Any one of these techniques may be used independently of the other two.) The insertion of prostaglandins in tylose paste into the cervical canal as pessaries are employed to induce labour without rupturing the membranes. It also precludes the use of intravenous infusion.

The effect of the management of labour on its length and on fetal and maternal mortality and morbidity has been reviewed elsewhere, widely publicised, but is now being reassessed.

The effect of the process on the mothers self-concept and on her mothering role has so far not been investigated. Further evaluation of its effects on the baby are also needed although some studies are already available (see Ch. 9). The very development of management techniques has arisen from, and expedited the improvement of, diagnosis of abnormality.

It is an everyday observation, reinforced by more precise data from experimental studies in social psychology, that the individual is susceptible to pressures to conformity (Asch 1956 and Sherif 1935). It is also clear that some people are more influential in exerting pressure on others. Numerical strength is important, as is high status and success, indeed the terms are almost synonymous with influence.

The medical profession have for many decades enjoyed high status and an influential position in the community.

Within the hospital setting they also have numerical strength. The likelihood is, therefore, that if a condition is defined in medical circles as abnormal it stands a good chance of being accepted as such. Obstetrics in the last decade has become extensively abnormalised and being in labour now not only necessitates going to hospital but in many cases having a special nurse in constant attendance (O'Driscoll 1975), a state of affairs usually associated with serious illness. It is likely that a proportion of normal women with normal pregnancies succumb to expectations. We suggest here the process by which this may occur. By defining labour as a medical event requiring hospital treatment and highly skilled surveillance, the general level of anxiety about it may be raised. There is evidence that pre-natal attitudes and anxieties have an effect on the length of labour and the incidence of complications (Engström et al. 1964, Davids & Devaultz 1962, Zemlick & Watson 1953). Crawford (1969) has suggested the mechanism by which fears and anxieties can affect the process of labour. As a result of anxiety adrenaline is secreted into the bloodstream, and this restricts the blood supply to, and contractions of, the uterus, Hawkins (1974) says 'The main effect of adrenaline on the pregnant human uterus is to depress both intensity and frequency of contractions . . . The action is accompanied by tachycardia and systolic hypertension and the utero placental circulation may be affected in an unpredictable manner with the production of fetal distress.' Crawford (1969) found that women who showed overt signs of anxiety at the onset of labour (expressed fear, high pulse rate, etc.) were more likely to develop problems related to uterine dysfunction and their infants to develop hypoxia. Uterine inertia is one of the problems which the active management of labour is designed to ameliorate however, O'Driscoll (1975) notes 'Active management ensures efficient uterine action'. The very prospect for some women of being actively managed however may interfere with the normal sequence of endocrine activity which leads to uterine efficiency. Hypertonic contractions do not always become more efficient even with the use of syntocinon and the possibility that psychological and biochemical events are counteracting each other deserves further exploration.

In so far as modern obstetrics increases anxieties it may

have exacerbated the very condition that it seeks to ameli-orate. A woman's admission to hospital and her loss of autonomy at the onset of labour invest the experience with a dimension of apprehension which through the consequent endocrine activity, depresses uterine function and increases the likelihood of a delay in labour and fetal distress. This in turn requires further intervention.

ACTIVE MANAGEMENT OF LABOUR

Debate in both public and medical press has expressed concern about both the short and long term effects of the active management of labour on mothers, their children and their families. It has also greatly affected the work of the midwife and her role in society.

Induction of labour in England in 1965 was estimated to have been performed in 15 per cent of deliveries and this rose to an estimated 40.7 per cent in 1974. There was a steady rise till the late 1970s. The DHSS Annual Report for 1975 found 'no cause for concern in the current use of induction tech-niques . . . in some cases there did appear to be a failure of communication between staff and their patients. . . . It was felt that many of the complaints about induction made by women reflected a deeper underlying dissatisfaction with the extent to which their emotional and psychological needs are being catered for in childbirth.' In the late 1970s rates started to fall and in 1980 an estimated 20 per cent of women in NHS beds were induced; 13.1 per cent had instrumental deliveries. Comparative figures for women in pay beds were 32 per cent and 24.2 per cent respectively (Macfarlane & Mugford 1986).

Amniotomy has to be followed by uterine stimulation if contractions do not ensue within a fairly short time. This process involves the midwife in close monitoring of both fetal and maternal conditions because the effects on mother and fetus of the artificially increased strength of contractions is not always predictable. Where epidural analgesia is adminis-tered the need for constant surveillance is increased as the mother is unaware of the strength of her uterine activity and the risk of hypotension is ever present.

It has been claimed that one of the advantages of the

induction and acceleration of labour is that 'it has created a situation where every woman in labour has a personal nurse . . . This personal contact provides invaluable support for morale and it also provides an opportunity for student nurses' (sic) 'and doctors to gain an insight into the human element of labour which they previously lacked', (O'Driscoll 1975).

It has always been a requirement of the Central Midwives Board (and now the National Boards for Nursing, Midwifery & Health Visiting), however, that no woman is left alone from the beginning of the second stage of labour until the end of the third stage (CMB 1962) and many have been attended throughout the first stage as well. The midwife, monitoring an actively managed labour, may feel that mechanical knowledge and ability is more relevant than human insight.

It is usually a student midwife or obstetric nurse who is required to stay with a woman during the course of a managed labour. She may be both young and inexperienced, obstetrically and generally and may be hard pressed to sustain either her patient or herself with relevant comfort and solace. For two people to have to maintain a relationship while segregated in a separate room for several hours, may be an entertaining and satisfying experience if they like each other. If they do not, or if there is some cause for embarrassment, it may be a great trial. The plight of a distraught student who acted as the special nurse for a patient with an intrauterine death for several hours, demands sympathy. It was not clear to her whether the patient was aware that her baby had died. Probably they dared not mention the topic foremost in their minds. Several hours at what is often a monotonous and repetitive task can be very dispiriting. Human beings are extremely bad at maintaining alert attentiveness in conditions of monotony (Mackworth 1950). Any member of staff should have the option of being relieved of such a duty after an hour or at most two.

This may seem to be contradicting our view of the midwife giving continuity of care. It would be very satisfactory if the midwife who had supervised the patient's antenatal care and education, and had come to know her well could be with her throughout her labour. The demands on trained staff however would be excessive, and it seems inevitable that the 'continuity role' must be more supervisory in the first stage, and allow staff in training to carry out this essential job of monitoring of blood pressure, fetal and maternal pulse and so on.

Let us consider the sequence of events during labour and the supportive skills the midwife can bring to them. Labour may begin spontaneously and the first stage may be well advanced before patient and midwife meet. If the patient has attended antenatal classes she and her husband may have decided beforehand whether he is going to stay for the birth of the baby, and they will have some information as to the likely course of events. Patients who have not attended antenatal preparatory classes may need some information at this stage, and both parents need some opportunity for discussion to decide whether the husband is to be present. The patient's fullest cooperation in the birth process is to be encouraged and she and her husband need to decide whether his presence will help. Husbands in the labour ward are encouraged in most hospitals, though the idea may be out of keeping with prevailing attitudes of some cultural groups and should not be insisted upon.

A considerable proportion of patients are admitted to hospital before labour starts spontaneously, with a view to induction. The unseemly position of lithotomy is unlikely to be reassuring, and patients need a proper explanation of the purpose of an amniotomy. A woman in a position appropriate for an artificial rupture of membranes is unlikely to be sufficiently relaxed to take in all that is said to her at the time by way of explanation. The midwife may do much to encourage her morale, not only by answering questions and providing information, but by assuring her that someone will always be close by, preferably before the procedure is carried out. Ideally the person in constant contact and attendance should be known to the patient. If the important 'continuity role' has been developed during the antenatal period the confidence of the patient is likely to be greatly enhanced. The knowledge that she is being cared for by someone who is aware of her development during the pregnancy will be reassuring. It is to the midwife that women must look to counteract the depersonalisation which accompanies much of modern obstetrics. To provide good continuity of care the midwife needs to

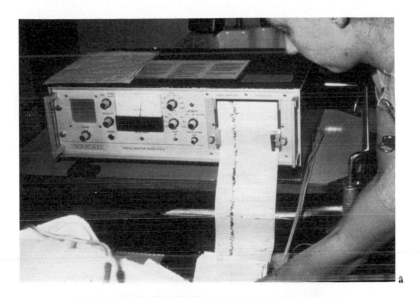

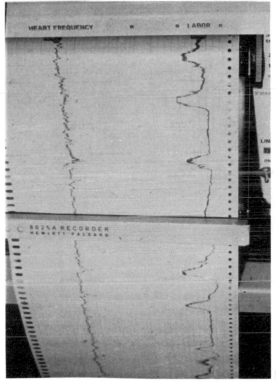

Figure 5.1a & b Progress of patient can be checked on monitoring apparatus rather than by personal examination

know something of the patient's hopes and fears, to be available not only to give information, but to listen. Confidences are only entrusted to those who are known and respected.

The progress of labour may be normal and natural and the patient free to walk around until late first or second stage of labour. When the labour is induced, accelerated, and monitored, movement is often restricted by the infusion and cardiotocograph. Some women in antenatal classes express their apprehension at the idea of being attached to machinery and being unable to get off the bed. There is a number of possible reasons for this. The control of bowel and bladder movement is very deeply ingrained by early training, as is a strong reticence about their activity. Complaints about not being able to get up to go to the lavatory must be one of the most common in all hospital patients. The return to infancy implied by soiling, or dependence on someone else to deal with these primitive needs, is a trauma not to be lightly dismissed. In addition many women in normal labour find walking about of some comfort. Physiologically it is a better position for facilitating childbirth than being flat on a bed.

Having to keep still on a bed emphasises the sickness or dependence role, while the monitoring apparatus may depersonalise the experience. Attention is divided between the patient on the bed and the machinery at her side (Figs. 5.1a & b). Her progress may be checked less by how she feels, more by the recording. Close attention to the paper record can provide the obstetrician with the information he needs. This can be acquired without a word to, or an examination of, the patient. It has been known that the recording apparatus was housed in a separate room from the patient so she could be monitored but left alone. This is inimical to the age-old view that the midwife is the person to be 'with the wife'.

BIRTH POSITION

The horizontal position for delivery is dictated by requirements of monitoring. It may not be the most efficient for either the mother or the fetus. The pelvic musculature is affected by position as is the blood supply to the baby. The position in which to give birth may be an aspect of a cultural tradition handed down from mother to daughter. In such a case it will have a significance beyond the immediate one of functional efficiency, and midwives should be prepared to respond sympathetically to mothers who want to be delivered in a squatting, standing or other unconventional position. The President of the Royal College of Midwives, Dorothy Webster, said at the College's annual meeting in 1982: 'There is a move towards less technology and more natural childbirth and we must give a lead by being ready and willing to adjust to these changes'. In so far as unconventional expectations about position for delivery are associated with mothers from ethnic minorities the midwife has a special responsibility. The health problems of particular minority groups do cause concern (e.g. rickets in Asian children) especially when associated with non-take-up of the services that are available. The experience a mother has of her treatment during childbirth will colour her view of how services are delivered, and may affect her family's willingness to use them in the future.

Any broad cultural group – English, Indian, Chinese etc. – has a variety of finer distinctions within it. An English woman's ideas about childbirth may vary according to her religion, social class and possibly the part of the country in which she grew up and so on. It is very desirable that health workers who deal with members of particular sects, cultural groups etc. should be acquainted as fully as possible with their customs and expectations. This will help avoid an unwitting conflict over – for example – birth position or presence of the husband at the birth.

Some patients express great satisfaction with hospital delivery. Women who have had difficult or very painful deliveries before may be reassured by the quality of technical achievement manifest in a modern labour ward. There may be a number of reasons why they have come to distrust human frailty – including their own. For others the mechanisation of a human experience is objectionable and alienating. The labour ward with its monitoring apparatus, stainless steel and impersonal purity is completely at odds with the homely test that has been made for the baby in the preceeding weeks (Fig. 5.2). The home is marked by symbols of personal taste

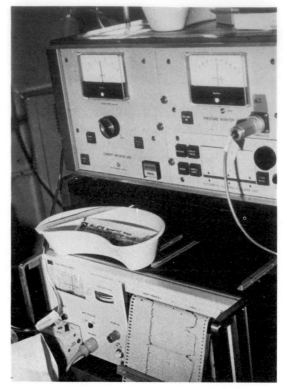

Figure 5.2 Technical apparatus of labour ward.

and individuality which gives it meaning. The hospital ward has a small area which can be given some personal meaning by photographs on the locker and the paraphernalia of interests and hobbies. The labour ward is purified of every personal symbol, with the permissable exception of a woman's wedding ring.

The midwife may be able to provide good help and support by recognising and responding to the important individual traits and motivations be they attractive or otherwise. Not all women are delighted at the prospect of producing a baby. Some are fearful, resentful, faced with the inevitability of labour and delivery. Very few women openly express hostility to the fetus about to be born, and negative statements about any aspect of having a baby are rarely heard in a maternity hospital: yet they must exist. Criticisms of the baby who is the wrong sex are perhaps an exception to this.

There are certainly strong social restrictions to the voicing of criticism. Dana Breen (1975) in her study of women having their first baby suggests that 'the discrepancy between what the woman experiences and what she is told she should be experiencing' can be a factor contributing to post natal depression. Perhaps most women are made to feel that they should be grateful (for all that is done for them) and joyful (with their new baby). What they may feel is resentment and anger (at not being able to do things their own way) and bitter or disappointed (at the birth and their new baby). Post-natal depression is an important problem which is discussed further in the next chapter. It might be to great advantage if the midwife can tolerate, or perhaps even facilitate, the expression of adverse feelings of a woman in labour. What many women fear is that such feelings are unusual, abnormal, and frightening. It cannot be urged too frequently that affection for a baby is largely learned and that no great alarm should arise over the expression of antipathetic feelings during labour, or even on first seeing the baby.

A patient who is immobile because she is attached to apparatus is bound to feel passive rather than active. Her movements, behaviour, progress in labour, her bodily sensations are constrained or initiated at the behest of someone else. She is passively expected to react to management by others, to follow instructions rather than determine the course of events for herself. This becomes more markedly the case for patients who have epidural analgesia. An increase in epidurals seem to be associated with an increase in instrumental delivery. The enormous motive power from within is reduced to a less efficient level. One woman we know had all her four healthy children at home. On every occasion she refused to call the midwife until the very last moment because 'I didn't want anyone to come and fiddle about with me'. Dana Breen (1975) found that the women 'who went through the experience of having a child with least difficulties, where those women who were able to feel themselves to be active, not only after the birth of the baby but also during pregnancy. Such a sense of initiation and activity is one which has often been denied women in our culture.' (Breen 1975). It is denied too to a large number of women who are managed during their labour. The midwife does need to use considerable tact and skill to help a woman in normal labour to retain her initiative and active integrity, and to restrain others with a more active approach to the problem.

PAIN RELIEF

Discussion of pain relief is done in some antenatal classes; but not all women attend these. There is often some need therefore to expand on the matter during labour. A few women attend relaxation classes and so successfully apply what they have learned that analgesics are not needed. There are rather few women who manage this. Some apply themselves diligently to exercises and breathing and go to pieces when the going gets rather rougher than they anticipated. They may feel ashamed at having lost control or frightened because they believe something abnormal is occurring. Others are ready to consider analgesics if necessary but want to know what risks to themselves and the baby are associated with each method. The acceleration of labour by oxytocic drugs of course makes contractions suddenly become stronger, and therefore women in accelerated labour are likely to require more pain relief. There is evidence that the analgesic given to the mother during labour does affect the infant. By making him drowsy and unresponsive the early mother – baby relationship may be more difficult to establish. Babies whose mothers have had barbiturates or pethidine suck with less vigour and perhaps because of that gain weight less well. They habituate more slowly, are more difficult to console and have more interuptions in their feeding (Brazelton 1973, Richards & Bernal 1973). Whether there are any long term consequences is not yet clear.

The subjective experience of pain has no direct relationship to the extent of physical trauma. There is much evidence that the experience of pain is affected by previous experiences and how well they are remembered, by the understanding we have of the cause of the pain and its consequences. Scott-Palmer and Skevington (1981) found that women who believed themselves to be in personal control of their lives experienced shorter labours with more intense pain per hour than those believing in the uncontrollability of events. Different cultures accord different kinds of significance to pain and these evaluations are learned during growing up. Animals reared in conditions where they experienced no hurtful stimuli appeared lacking in a proper appreciation of pain when they were grown up. They made no effort to get away from a flame, showed little evidence of pain when pricked, (Thompson & Melzack 1956).

Sportsmen often sustain serious injury on the playing field and fail to notice it till the game is over. Soldiers in combat have been oblivious to extensive trauma. Any situation that attracts attention away from the source of the pain tends to reduce the experience of it. Hypnosis works on this basis. Hypnosis is a trance like state in which the subject's attention is focused intensely on the hypnotist while attention to other stimuli is markedly diminished. A few people are sufficiently susceptible to undergo surgery without anaesthesia. For some others hypnosis can reduce the amount of analgesic required. Morgan et al (1984) in a study based on replies from 632 mothers delivered at Queen Charlotte's Hospital found strong support for the statement: 'Having a sympathetic midwife to help mothers throughout labour is more important than all treatment for pain relief'.

Emotional support has already been referred to as effective in reducing pain (see p. 58). Attention is diverted from the source of the pain and the personal contact reduces fear. Anyone who has suffered prolonged pain regards it as an evil, and harmful in itself.

Yet the positive aspects of pain as a biological warning system are well recognised. Any experienced midwife knows the element of pain relief there is in the confidence a patient has in her. This effective confidence is not established quickly, and the need for it gives added point to our proposition that the effective midwife needs to maintain a continuity role with the patient.

The husband in the labour ward if he is suitably motivated and informed may well be able to provide vital confidence and support. Henneborn and Cogan (1975) have studied the effects of husbands at the delivery (Fig. 5.3). They found that the presence of husbands (who had attended antenatal

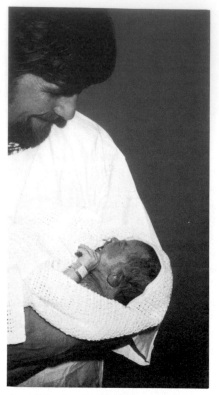

Figure 5.3 Husband participating in the labour ward.

classes) had a positive effect on their wives' reported feelings of pain, and there was a decreased use of medication. For the hospital delivery the husband too is on strange territory, and he will be much less able to help his wife if his own position is ambiguous by his being made to feel unwelcome. Some people have argued that husbands might lay claim to the right to be in the labour ward. If he is there, the wise midwife can make full use of his consoling potential by assuring him of a welcome, making it clear to him how he can help and what he can do. If he has a clearly defined role he is likely to live up to it. Only when he does not know what is expected of him, is he likely to get in the way, or faint, as some of his critics have claimed! This might well be a mismanagement of a valuable resource. He also needs help and considerate support as it is often as difficult to watch suffering as to experience it. There are various ways in which preparatory antenatal education is organised. It was found (Cambell & Worthington 1981) that explicit structured training for expectant fathers was much more effective than unstructured discussion as a preparation for helping their partners during labour. The mothers too felt more confident with the assistance they received from men who had had specific instruction.

Episiotomy and instrumental delivery have increased together with the increase in the control of labour. Both of these activities, like amniotomy and administration of oxytocic drugs, have as their rationale, the acceleration of delivery. An increase in instrumental delivery may be associated upon the increase in the use of epidural analgesic often needed because of the increased strength of contractions in accelerated labour. Epidural analgesia, as well as deadening the painful experience of uterine contractions reduces or removes the urgency for women to make expulsive effort. In the study by Morgan referred to above, 50 per cent agreed that 'an epidural block is the best sort of pain relief in labour'; 20 per cent disagreed.

The advantages and disadvantages of these practices have been hotly debated by a variety of interested groups. Obstetricians, paediatricians, midwives, psychologists, women's movements, patients' associations, especially those which concern themselves with the services available to pregnant and parturient women, have all expressed their views. The debate is basically an ideological one. Those who favour control and acceleration argue that a proportion of women, especially those having first babies, are going to have abnormal labours and it is impossible to predict in advance those who are at risk. Caution therefore demands that all patients be treated as high risk. As it is during the labour and delivery that emergencies arise, the more speedily mother and baby are separated under conditions of maximum surveillance, the better. Those who take the opposite view regard childbirth as a natural phenomenon in which a myriad of factors orchestrate in a finely balanced, but as yet poorly understood way. Proponents of this view believe that a spontaneous delivery by a healthy, self-confident, and reasonably happy woman cannot be improved upon, and that the job of the maternity services is to enhance the woman's health, self-confidence and happiness. This they claim can best be achieved by encouraging her autonomy, providing moral support and eschewing all meddling (Kloosterman 1975).

There has been, of course, a dramatic improvement in maternal and perinatal mortality rates but it would be a mistake to attribute this entirely to interventionist policies of current obstetrics in the United Kingdom.

Home confinement is still common in Holland. In 1984 approximately one third of all confinements were at home. The rate is lower in large towns where there is a hospital within easy reach, and higher in less populated parts.

On first booking – with a family doctor, midwife or obstetrician – a first selection is made in the light of a list of medical indications. 15 per cent of all women have a 'primary medical indication' for hospital delivery under the supervision of an obstetrician. In the absence of a primary medical indication the woman may decide whether to have her baby at home or in hospital. During the course of pregnancy if a 'secondary medical indication' arises she will be obliged to have a hospital delivery. Damstra-Wijmenga (1984) has reported on the outcome for 1692 women (i.e. 99.3 per cent of total births) in 1981 in Groningen. 56 per cent chose to be delivered by a midwife and 42.4 per cent were actually so delivered. 23.4 per cent chose home delivery and 19 per cent were actually delivered there. As parity increased, the option on home confinement was more frequently used.

In a number of cases disorders developed during the course of the pregnancy and during labour, which required referral to an obstetrician. These were lowest among women who had chosen home delivery, as was infant morbidity. In Holland the proportion of instrumental deliveries is smaller than that in any other western country; maternal and perinatal mortality rates are among the lowest in the world. In seeking an explanation Damstra-Wijmenga comments: 'The fact that in a hospital or maternity clinic the very surroundings and equipment may give rise to iatrogenic complications is apparently overlooked' in the arguments about the increasing medicalisation of childbirth. A study in England and Wales in 1979 (Campbell et al 1982) showed that perinatal mortality was much higher in home deliveries than the national average (24.3 as compared with 14.6 per thousand). Further analysis of the figures for England and Wales showed them to be strongly influenced by the high proportion of illegitimate births.

Perinatal and infant mortality rates are sensitive indicators of social conditions. The midwife in the labour ward has, however, to work within the constraints of the immediate situation, where these wider considerations may seem remote. Patients who are drowsy through medication are not necessarily unaware of what is said or done around them, nor are their husbands. They sometimes cannot, often do not, make it plain that they can both see and hear. It is unlikely to do the patient a service to openly comment upon episiotomy or haemorrhage or to display to view implements for instrumental delivery. Not only is she likely to be frightened unnecessarily but any misunderstanding can undermine her confidence in the staff, which may subsequently have serious consequences.

CAESARIAN SECTION

Some women experience an instrumental delivery as a great disappointment, and the rise in the Caesarian section rate is a matter of concern for this and other reasons. 8.8 per cent of all deliveries in England and Wales in 1980 were by Caesarian section. The social (as well as the clinical) consequences for parents and babies may be considerable. The establishment of breast feeding is more difficult, postnatal stay in hospital is longer (17.4 per cent had wound infection (Moir et al 1984), and one enquiry suggests that parents feel less positive about babies resulting from a Caesarian section (Garel & Kaminski 1904). On return home the mother is recovering from a major operation which makes return to normal family life more difficult and is also likely to create extra expense for the family in the form of home help and formula feeding.

Probably the most rewarding experience for both parents and midwife is the occasion when the mother retains sufficient consciousness and control to actively participate in and watch the birth of the baby. This can be an ecstatic experience. Aidan McFarlane (1977) has recorded the conversations between parents, baby and staff at and immediately following normal deliveries. Against the background of realism with crying baby, metallic instruments, blood and dirty linen they speak of a profound pleasure. The baby is inspected minutely, discussed and put in a relationship to various members of the family. 'Got my nose and ears', 'big feet', 'look at his hair', 'to be known as Kirsty', 'you're not a Cameron at all', 'She's lovely. I thought she'd be all mauve and crinkly' 'Well it will suit your Mum won't it?' The opportunity for the mother and father to look at and handle the baby within seconds of his birth gives great pleasure (Fig. 5.4). They can assure themselves of his good health and take pride in their achievement, and have their first conversation with the new member of the family. Many mothers have complained that their babies are taken away after the birth and they may not see them again for several hours. If the mother was not conscious for the delivery she may spend hours worrying about his very existence.

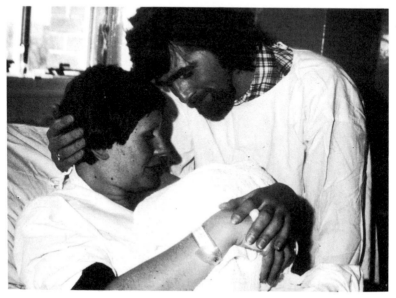

Figure 5.4 Mother and father handling baby immediately after birth.

THE UNSUPPORTED MOTHER

The unsupported mother at the antenatal clinic has been discussed. When she is in labour she is likely to need special care and attention from the midwife. The schoolgirl mother is a subject of particular concern. Scarcely out of childhood herself she may be the focal point of many problems. Not infrequently from a disrupted family she may be blamed, abused or ignored by her upset parents on account of the pregnancy. She may be advised, cajoled or bullied by a cacophony of voices not necessarily with her or the baby's welfare as priorities. Some young pregnant girls can easily be overwhelmed by their mothers who plan to take over the baby and treat him as their own. The grafting of the new baby on to the end of an established family may be satisfactory where it is done with affection, tact and consideration for the baby and the true mother. There are families however where this has set the scene for disasterous confusion of relationships. The child is often brought up believing his mother to be his sister, his uncle to be his brother, his grandmother his mother so on. The discovery of the truth of these relationships can be disruptively distressing. The realignment of such close relationships implies a major realignment of the self, and may herald the onset of psychotic behaviour (Gibbens 1963).

THE BABY FOR ADOPTION

A woman who has decided during the pregnancy that the baby is to be adopted will also, it is hoped, have had the opportunity of discussing the implications of this decision (see p. 52–4). Mothers who are separated from their babies involuntarily or whose babies die, suffer anxicty, depression or grief. A voluntary giving away of the baby involves more personal responsibility and possibly a stronger feeling of guilt. Children sometimes go to inordinate lengths to try to find their lost parents. They feel that they are incomplete unless they can find the people who gave them their beginning. This will become a highly complex matter with further advances – technically and in the extent of application – in the practice of artificial fertilisation (see p. 33). Without knowledge of their parents, people often feel they are unable to answer the question 'Who am I?' to their satisfaction. It is now legally possible and permissible for adopted children to trace their biological parents. This is likely to have a considerable impact on attitudes to adoption as the ill-begotten child may resurface after eighteen years.

When the baby is born there is the question of whether the mother should see, or hold her baby. The longer mother and baby are in contact the greater the wrench of separation when it comes. Some women decide firmly not to see the baby at all, and keep to their plan. Some make the decision and change their minds at the birth. Some never make any hard and fast decision and, of course, some who have planned adoption all through the pregnancy change their minds after the birth.

Folklore and myth abound with stories of revenge exacted, peace restored, old scores settled by the emergence in adulthood of children abandoned, given away or believed dead. The recurrence of such themes shows how feelings of guilt, hope or grief remain unresolved and emerge in symbolic form in such stories as Oedipus Rex, The Winter's Tale, Snow White and many others. The child who is the focus of suspicion, embarrassment or threat may be put out of sight but not out of mind. We have been unable to find any systematic study of women who have had their babies adopted. The recent change in the law relating to adopted children adds another variable to be taken into account when coming to a decision.

Mothers used to be obliged to look after their babies for six weeks before placing them for adoption and the overt purpose was to give them time to make a considered decision. Another six weeks follows before the court order can be made. Many undoubtedly became attached to their babies in that time and either changed their minds or suffered considerably at the parting. It seemed to many people kinder to let a woman avoid becoming really fond of her baby by not having contact. How far this new legislation will affect decisions at birth remains to be seen. A midwife who inevitably becomes involved in discussion and decisions on the issue should be aware of the complex psycho-social issues involved.

We hear a lot about the need to support the family against all the insidious pressures that are suspected of weakening it. What goes on during labour and delivery may have effects on the way the mother sees herself – active or passive – directed or autonomous – in control or the victim of circumstances. The midwife has a clear and influencial role to play, in helping the mother to adapt effectively and to sustain a positive vigorous attitude to herself, her baby and her family.

REFERENCES

Asch, S. E. (1956) Studies of independence and submission to group pressure. *Psychological Monographs*, 70 (416).

Association for the Improvement of the Maternity Services. (1975) *Quarterly Newsletter*, March, p. 7.

Brazelton, T. B. (1973) Effect of prenatal drugs on the behaviour of the neonate. *American Journal of Psychiatry*, 126 pp 1261–1266.

Breen, Dana. (1975) *Birth of a First Child*. London: Tavistock Publications.

Cambell, A. & Worthington E. L. (1981) A comparison of two methods of training husbands to assist their wives with labour and delivery. *Journal of Psychosomatic Research*, 25 (6) pp 557–563.

Campbell, R., MacDonald Davies I. & Macfarlane, A. (1982) Perinatal mortality and place of delivery. *Population Trends*, 28.

CMB Handbook 25th Edition 1962 p 59.

Crawford, Mary I. (1969) Psychological & Behavioural Clues to Disturbances in Childbirth. Columbia University Dissertation. Available in the UK in *Dissertation Abstracts*, 29 (7-B) p 2504.

Damstra-Wijmenga, S. M. I. (1984) Home confinement: the positive results in Holland. *Journal of the Royal College of General Practitioners*, 34 pp 425–430.

Davids, A. & Devault, S. (1962) Maternal Anxiety during Pregnancy and Childbrith Abnormalities. *Psychosomatic Medicine*, 24 (5) pp 464–470.

Annual Report of the Chief Medical Officer for 1975 (1976) DHSS. London: HMSO.

Engstrom, L., Afgeiterstam, G., Holmberg, N. G. & Uhrus, K. (1964) A prospective study of the relationship between psycho-social factors and the course of pregnancy and delivery. *Journal of Psychosomatic Research*, 8 pp 151–155.

Garel, M. & Kaminski, M. (1984) Review of evaluative studies on Caesarian section. EEC Workshop, Brussels March 14 16.

Gibbens, T. C. N. (1963) *Psychiatric Studies of Borstal Lads*. Oxford: O.U.P.

Hawkins, D. F. (1974) The pharmacology of the pregnant human uterus. In *Obstetric Therapeutics*, Ed. Hawkins, D. F., p 31. London: Balliere.

Henneborn, W. J. & Cogan, R. (1975) The effect of husband participation on reported pain and the probability of medication during labour and birth. *Journal of Psychosomatic Research*, 1i. pp 215–222.

Kitzinger, Sheila. (1971) Woman on the Delivery Table. In *Woman on Woman*, Ed. Laing, Margaret. London: Sidgwick & Jackson.

Kloosterman, G. J. (1975) Obstetrics in the Netherlands – a survival or a challenge? (Paper presented to the Meeting on Problems in Obstetrics

organised by the Medical Information Unit of Spastics' Society at
Tunbridge Wells.)

McFarlane, Aidan. (1977) *Psychology of Childbirth*. London: Fontana Open
Books.

Macfarlane, A. & Mugford, M. (1986) An epidemic of Caesarians? *Maternal
and Child Health*. February pp 38–42.

Mackworth, N. H. (1950) Researches in the Measurement of Human
Performance. *M.R.C.* Special Report Series. No. **268**. London: HMSO.

Mead, Margaret. (1950) *Male and Female*. London: Victor Gollanz.

Moir, B. M., Hulton, R. & Thompson, J. (1984) Wound infection after
Caesarian Section. *Journal of Hospital Infection*, 5 pp 359–370.

Morgan, B. M., Bulpitt, C. J. Clefton, P. & Lewis, P. J. (1984) The
consumers' attitude to obstetric care. *British Journal of Obstetrics and
Gynaecology*, **91** pp 624–628.

O'Driscoll, Kieran. (1975) Active Management of Labour. *Midwife, Health
Visitor & Community Nurse*, **11** pp 146–148.

Revans, R. W. (1964) Standards for morale: cause and effect in hospitals.
Oxford: Oxford University Press for the Nuffield Provincial Hospital
Trust.

Richards, M. P. M. & Bernal, J. F. (1972) An observational study of mother-
infant interaction. In *Ethological Studies of Child Behaviour*. Ed. Burton-
Jones, N. London: Cambridge University Press.

Scott-Palmer, J. & Skevington, S. M. (1981) Pain during childbirth and
mensturation: A study of locus of control. *Journal of Psychosomatic
Research*, **25** (3) pp 151–155.

Sherif, M. (1935) A Study of some Social Factors in Perception. *Archives of
Psychology*, **27** (187) pp 5, 17, 34, 41.

Thompson, W. R. & Melzack, R. (1956) Early Environment. *Scientific
American*, **194** pp 38–42.

Zemlick, M. J. & Watson, D. (1953) Maternal attitudes of acceptance and
rejection during and after pregnancy. *American Journal of
Orthopsychiatry*, **23** pp 570–584.

6

Boy or girl

'It's a girl'. 'It's a boy'. These words are the first spoken at
many deliveries. Friends and relatives are informed, telephone wires buzz with *son, daughter,* and cards in either blue
or pink are despatched. Interest in the sex of the new baby
takes second place only to a concern for its health.

IMPORTANCE OF SEXUAL IDENTITY IN SOCIAL ENCOUNTERS

At all social encounters the sexual identity of the other person
is a matter of primary concern. Birth is the first social
encounter and ends several months of speculation about the
baby's appearance, personality and sex. During the pregnancy
and especially during the final weeks when the fetus is
constantly making its presence felt, mothers spend a lot of
time thinking about their baby, how they will look after it,
what it will be called, where it will sleep, and so on. An
important part of this forward planning is the sex of the child.
Some have strong preferences or premonitions, while some
are unconcerned about whether they have a boy or girl.

ANTENATAL ADJUSTMENTS

The antenatal period is one in which old established relation-ships are reviewed in the knowledge that a new relationship has to be made. If a baby girl is contemplated the mother may think of her as having some of the important characteristics and personality of her own mother or sister, and in her imag-ination, relive some of the relationships she has had with them. There are numerous indications that the course of pregnancy is characterised by changes in a woman's mood and behaviour. Some of these serve all important functions in helping her to adapt to her impending new role of mother-hood. Taking on a new role means modifying already existing ones. A woman may, on one day imagine herself with a boy baby and wonder how such a child will fit in with the family. She may consider how her own mother and father will feel about him and how he will affect her relationships with other close relatives and friends. The idea of having a little boy can arouse feelings that have been associated with her father, husband, brother or other important male figures in her life. On another day, the coming baby can be thought of as a little girl, and a correspondingly female set of relation-ships, feelings and ideas will be experienced. This review period may serve some important preparatory function.

As pregnancies are subject to increasing surveillance some careful enquiry into the effects of investigations, inter-ferences, and the provision of information, on the psycho-logical functioning of the mother is needed. Many mothers, having had an amniocentesis, vigourously reject the idea of knowing the sex of their child. Giving the mother information about the sex of the fetus may limit the mental explorations that are undertaken. We can only speculate as to how the thinking, fantasies, and day dreams of pregnancy affect the maternal response when the baby arrives. What is fairly certain, however, is that babies even before they are born are rarely thought of as neuter. Assigning a sex to the fetus may vary from day to day or it may be consistently 'Jane' or 'Robert' from fairly early in the pregnancy.

Producing a baby has much in common with roulette. Innumerable chance factors affect the outcome, and much of the zest is in the excitement and anticipation before the pointer comes to rest. If accurate predictions can be made, enthusiasm wanes. Extreme predictability and extreme novelty are both avoided by human beings so far as possible. The one is boring and the other frightening. Enough novelty to maintain interest, but not so much as to induce a feeling of insecurity, provides an agreeable situation for most of us. Sexual identity is so central to personality, that to know the sex of the baby before it is born may increase the boredom of the gestation period. This is clearly an area where speculation could, with profit, give way to some objective findings.

PREFERENCES OF PARENTS

In any society where preferences of parents for boys or girls has been recorded, the result is consistently predictable. Boys have been, and are, universally more highly valued. There may be a good economic origin for this. In conditions where the population growth constantly threatens to outstrip resources, boys bring to the family the possibility of more labour and increased resources, whereas girls in addition to their potential for work, bring the possibility of more children. There are innumerable sayings from all over the world which testify to the low regard in which girls have been held, for example 'May you have a hundred sons'; 'When a girl is born the walls weep'. A letter of Lady Frances Hatton to her husband in 1678 after the birth of their third daughter, reads, 'I am sure you will love it though it be a girl and I trust to God that I may live to bring you boys'. Until about a hundred years ago the Neapolitans would hang a small black flag from the window if a girl was born. This saved the neighbours the embarrassment of making enquiries.

The Agricultural and Industrial Revolutions, by greatly increasing resources, reduced the pressure of population, and contraception in advanced countries has further reduced the problem. Attitudes, however, are passed from one generation to another, and can take a long time to change. A study in America in 1957 showed that the first choice of family for potential parents, is to have one boy and one girl. The second choice was to have two boys (Clare & Kiser 1957).

Parents who already had one child and were asked what sex

of child they would have liked, modified their choice in favour of the already existing child. Husbands and wives of 173 families with a boy, and 192 families with a girl, gave the following replies (see Fig. 6.1). There is a marked tendency for parents to prefer a child of their own sex. The proportion of parents claiming no preference is also significantly higher when they have a girl. It is also plain that parents were more inclined to say they actually wanted the sex of child they had. It is more than likely that some of these parents changed their minds about their preference for a boy or girl after the baby was born.

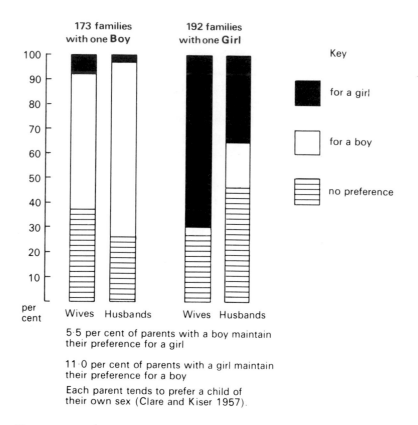

5·5 per cent of parents with a boy maintain their preference for a girl

11·0 per cent of parents with a girl maintain their preference for a boy

Each parent tends to prefer a child of their own sex (Clare and Kiser 1957).

Figure 6.1 Stated preference of those parents who already have either a boy or girl.

A case was reported in 1979 (Dove & Blow) of a pregnant woman, pregnant for the sixth time, who threatened to kill both herself and the baby should it be a girl. 'The uses to which amniocentesis may be put are wider than the medical purposes for which it was devised' the report points out. Although the final decision on abortion is a medical one, this particular case raised the issue of abortion on demand with the 'complex legal ethical and moral issues associated with it'.

There are in the urban industrial societies fairly strong pressures on parents to be good parents to both girls and boys. Strong personal preferences or dislikes are unlikely, therefore, to be acted upon. The mother who rejects her baby initially on account of its *wrong* sex, may need some very special help, but there are two things which ought to be remembered on the favourable side of this worrying situation. One is that affection of a mother for her child has a large learned component, and that if the mother can be supported by someone she trusts, the rejection may give way to a feeling of acceptance and affection. The other is that culturally there is now very much less discrimination against females, and also the distinctions between the sex roles have considerably blurred. Behaviour, attitudes and interests of boys and girls, men and women, overlap to an extent that was not possible in Victorian society for example. In societies where the sex roles are rigorously defined many people find their personality in conflict with the expectations others have of them. Florence Nightingale retreated to bed and invalidism to defend herself from the demands and expectations that her mother and sister had of her, that she should comply with the upper class female role of futile gentility. George Elliott and the Bronte Sisters wrote as men, because being intelligent or well-informed was incompatible with the female role at the time. Today boys and girls both play cricket and learn to cook, plan careers, go to parentcraft classes. In short, for both boys and girls, the range of acceptable behaviour is wider perhaps than ever before in any society. Although girls play cricket they play it less, and perhaps less well, than boys. Similarly, boys cook less than girls. There are attitudes, interests, apitudes and behaviour that are found more frequently in one of the sexes than the other.

MALE AND FEMALE PERSONALITY 'TYPES'

Innumerable psychological studies of men and women, boys and girls in USA and UK testify to the fact that there is a *modal* (most often occurring) personality for male and female. Males are more often aggressive, assertive, task orientated, ambitious: females are more often submissive, good with personal relationships, conformist, and verbal. Environmentalists have tended to explain such differences as a result of differential socialisation. Boys and girls are treated differently so they behave differently. The stories children usually hear present the girls as passive, sweet, and submissive, for example: Snow White, Rapunzel, Cinderella, and the boys as active, searching and dominant, for example: Tarzan, Lochinvar and Prince Charming. Boys and girls from babyhood are generally treated differently, have different activities which they are expected to imitate, and are encouraged to develop in different ways. The observations made by anthropologists of primitive cultures show that there is no inevitability about the development of male and female roles, such as exist in our society. Margaret Mead (1933) describes three tribes, the Mundugamoor, the Arapesh and the Tchambuli. Both male and female Mundugamoor behave in ways which we might describe as characteristic of males; both male and female Arapech have many qualities which in our society are connected with being female and, amongst the Tchambuli appropriate role behaviour is rather the reverse of our own. That is the women are more economically active and dominant, the men more submissive and retiring.

It is usually assumed that the physiological function is more or less fixed, and the environment may provide or withhold opportunities for its expression or development. There is some evidence, however, to show that environmental factors can alter endocrine activity. For example, aggressive responses are known to be related to male hormone levels. The defeat of a male rhesus monkey by another male, is followed by a rapid fall in his blood testosterone level, ensuring that his next encounter will be less aggressive. Adult rats who are handled in babyhood have a different autonomic and endocrine response to physical trauma and fear, from those who are not handled in babyhood (Levine 1961).

The smooth running of society depends, to a large extent, on the fact that most people do what is expected of them. An experiment in which teachers were given the intelligence test scores of the children in their class showed how well the test scores predicted achievements. The only disconcerting feature was that the scores were muddled up so that the teachers had in fact been misled. They expected a child with a high score to do well and one with a low score to do badly. Interaction between teachers and children was such as to bring this about. The point we are making is that many traits and characteristics that are thought of as *fixed* may in fact be changeable, if not fluid (Rosenthal & Jacobson 1966).

DIFFERENCES DURING PREGNANCY AND LABOUR WITH BOY AND GIRL BABIES

In a study of over 52 000 singleton deliveries over six years in Aberdeen it has been found that boy babies were delivered at earlier gestations than girls, and this difference was not due to induction or Caesarian section. In normal presentations girl babies were much more likely to deliver spontaneously, though female babies are more likely to be breech presentations. Pathological conditions (e.g. eclampsia) are more common in women carrying boy babies (Hall & Carr-Hill 1982).

DIFFERENCES BETWEEN NEWBORN GIRLS AND BOYS

At present little is known with any precision about the way in which newborn boys differ from newborn girls. Girls are smaller and lighter although neurologically more mature. More boys are asphyxiated at birth and they are more susceptible to disease. How far this susceptibility affects brain development, and therefore behaviour, has yet to be explored. Indeed little is known about the way specific neonatal problems affect development of personality and behaviour. Certainly the general picture is that boys start at a disadvantage physically. A study by Moss (1967) suggests how biological and social factors may interact together. Boy babies cry more, perhaps because they are physically less strong and mature, and at three weeks of age their mothers pick them up more. This behaviour is gradually reversed. With year-old children there is more close physical contact between mothers and daughters. It is possible that mothers become less responsive to insistent demands. Baby girls are more sensitive to tactile stimulation and to pain, but boys have better visual acuity.

Although there are a few sex differences at birth, the majority of dimensions on which infants differ show no observable sex differences. Girls are not more cuddly, boys are not more active, and so on. Babies in general vary in these and other behaviours but not on the basis of their sex. Work by Thomas et al. (1964) suggests that differences in temperament are the most important factors in enduring patterns of behaviour.

SEXUAL AND GENDER IDENTITY

There are, it is plain, traits and characteristics which are more commonly found in women, and others more commonly found in men. The influence of biological sex development on these characteristics varies. It is useful, therefore, to distinguish between sexual identify and gender identity. Sexual identify depends upon the possession of a male or female reproductive system. The large majority of biological males also feel masculine and behave as such. Biological females generally display feminine characteristics, so that their sexual and gender identity are consonant. Some little girls are described as tomboys, and women as having a masculine outlook; similarly the behaviour and attitudes of some men are more feminine. Gender identity is concerned with a wide range of attitudes, interests, preferences, ways of thinking, social behaviour and feelings. There are two possibilities only for sex identity (with the abnormal intersex condition making a rare third). Gender identity can range over a continuum from very masculine to very feminine.

PRENATAL SEXUAL DEVELOPMENT

At birth it is not usually difficult to determine whether the baby is a boy or girl. The judgement is normally made after inspection of the external genitalia. During the embryonic and fetal stages normal sexual development depends upon a number of factors. The human female has 23 pairs of chromosomes, one pair of which is, by convention, called the XX chromosomes – the male has 22 pairs and two unmatched ones, the X and Y chromosomes. The chromosome make up of the embryo is determined at conception and, providing the normal sequence of events occurs, the cell with XX chromosomes in the nucleus will grow to be a girl, and the cell with XY chromosomes to be a boy. Early embryonic development is the same for both sexes. Differentiation depends on an appropriate balance between the hormones androgen and oestrogen. Gonadal sex involving development of either ovaries or testes, is another essential feature of normal sexual development, and this is associated with the fourth factor, the internal reproductive system, and fifth the development of either the penis or vulva. There are five major biological jigsaw pieces which go to the making of boy or girl. They are chromosomes, hormones, gonads, internal reproductive system and external genitalia. Normally all these features, which together determine the sex of the infant, are consistent with each other, and sexual diagnosis is made on the basis of one of them, namely the external genitalia.

Very rarely the appearance of the genitalia may belie other parts of the reproductive system, or they may be neither clearly male nor female. The condition of Intersexuality is fortunately uncommon. There are a wide variety of aetiological factors which can contribute to intersexuality, and by the time the infant is born an anomalous stage in development has had an irreversible effect. Treatment is therefore directed to ameliorating a permanent condition.

INTERSEXUALITY: THE IMPORTANCE OF GENDER

Authorities on the subject are generally agreed that there is no one feature by which sex can be diagnosed, and that an attempt to diagnose the *true* sex, in a case of intersexuality, is mistaken. Initial efforts have to be directed towards helping the parents in their decision about how the child shall be reared – as a boy or as a girl. After the birth investigations are likely to be carried out in order to assemble a picture of chromosomal, biochemical, and anatomical features of the baby. The assessment of the sexual status of the child is complicated by considerations of possible developments at puberty. The decision about the sex to which the child shall be assigned, cannot wait until puberty. The parents cannot treat their child as neuter, and to be uncertain whether to treat it as a boy or girl is to invite psychosocial difficulties.

John Money of John Hopkins Hospital has followed up and reported on the gender identity of four intersex babies. All four were genetic females with hormonal activity which had induced a hypertrophied clitoris looking like a penis. One was assigned as a girl and reared as such, and one as a boy. The other two were assigned only provisionally – one as a girl, one as a boy. The psychosexual development of the first two was in accord with their assigned sex. The one assigned provisionally as a girl was ambivalent about her gender identity and wanted to be confirmed in her feminine role. The boy provisionally assigned was similarly ambivalent and wanted to be confirmed in his masculine role. Recourse to a study involving only four children may give an oversimplified view, but there does seem to be a high level of agreement amongst researchers and practitioners dealing with the problem of intersexuality, that the sex in which the child is reared carries the greatest weight. That is, for normal psychosocial functioning, what matters is that feelings, attitudes, interests, ideas about the self, aspirations and ambitions should be consistently masculine or consistently feminine. As these aspects of psychic development depend on learning, it is important that the people from whom the child will learn are consistent in their own behaviour and attitudes. Money takes the view that experience in the first three years of life is overwhelming importance in determining gender identity.

The parents will be the primary determinants of the child's gender role. If the baby is treated as a little boy, given boy's toys to play with and encouraged in boyish interests, he will develop a masculine gender role. A baby treated as a little girl, with pretty dresses to wear, an encouragement in feminine pursuits and interests, will develop a feminine gender role. Medical advisors would consider the extent of hormone support and the complexities of reconstructive surgery which would be necessary to promote one or the other role. It must be emphasised that the aim of any treatment and support is not to *make* the child either male or female in the physiological sense, but to make it possible for him or her to live a normal life free from the psychological difficulties associated with ambiguous sexuality.

In the last few years there have been a few well publicised *sex change* cases. These expose to public scrutiny the painful dilemma of people whose gender and sex role are incompatible. To have a body of one sex but the feeling, interests and aspirations of the other, is to live in a state of recurring, if not constant, conflict. Therapeutic endeavours are always directed to remodelling the sex organs or influencing the secondary sex characteristics of the body to accord with the psychic structure.

THE MIDWIFE'S ROLE IN HELPING PARENTS WHEN A SEXUALLY ANOMALOUS BABY IS BORN

It is very important for the midwife to look carefully at the first examination of the baby, as any deviation from the normal should be noted, as it may mean that there are more internal abnormalities than external. Also, if the baby has a hypospadias it may need surgical treatment before school age, when it could be a social handicap. The midwife caring for the mother and baby whose sexual status is ambiguous has a variety of problems with which to grapple. A very rare form of intersexuality (adrenogenital syndrome) is associated with a condition requiring early diagnosis and treatment, as the excess adrenal hormones can lead to early death. With other conditions it may be considered medically advisable for corrective surgery to be done fairly early in life. In either of these cases the parents are faced with problems similar to those discussed in Chapter 4, about the ill or handicapped baby. Here we will discuss problems arising specifically from the baby's sexual anomaly.

There will be some delay while investigations are undertaken before any discussion about practicalities of the baby's upbringing can be embarked upon. Meanwhile relatives and friends will be anxious to know whether a girl or boy has been born, and this may be a painful difficulty in presenting the new baby to its siblings. This period of suspense can only add to the distress of the parents. There may be a number of accessory worries which parents are likely to harbour. They may fear for the general health of their baby or wonder whether it will be of normal intelligence. A common reaction in any such adversity is to look for somewhere to put the blame, and a mother in particular may be additionally distressed by finding some defect, real or imagined, in herself or her actions. Questions of the child's eventual sexual capabilities and fertility may also arise.

Sex and gender roles pervade deeply into many aspects of psychosocial functioning. Presented with a baby whose sex has not been assigned means that the parents are confused as to how to behave towards it. Mother-with-son behaves in important ways differently from mother-with-daughter. Gender assignation being so important socially, most people have strong feelings on the subject; some are repulsed by aberrant sexuality, and presumably no one would positively chose it for their child.

The midwife's role in the period following the birth, and before a considered medical opinion can be offered, is a supportive one. There will be many questions and problems which arise and cannot be answered. There are a number of studies done in general hospitals which show that the patients facing the most traumatic experiences have the least social contact with nursing staff. The natural response to a painful or embarrassing dilemma is to avoid it if possible. The mother of an intersex baby may be much comforted by finding that there is someone who can talk with her, and perhaps share some of the difficulties that arise in handling an intersex baby, and in dealing with relatives. It is fortunately unlikely that any midwife will have the opportunity of learning much from experience, as the condition is relatively rare. Ambiguity has to be tolerated for a time, by everyone closely concerned with the baby. This means that the midwife is in no position to advise the parents and, knowing this, she may feel inhibited in her discourse with the mother. This is perhaps a situation in which a parent will ask direct questions, not with the expection of receiving an answer, but in the hope that someone will have the time and skill to listen sympathetically to how she views the problem.

The general public are very much better informed about medical matters than they were a few years ago. One consequence of this is a more general acceptance of the idea that medical and nursing professions do not know all the answers. To say 'we just don't know' is not a reflection of personal failure but an acknowledgement that medical science has not yet made progress in that particular direction. 'I don't know' may, of course, indicate a personal inadequacy as it may mean 'the information is available but I am not acquainted with it'. A midwife can always undertake to try to find out. It may be quite rewarding to enquire of the parents what they know and what their ideas are.

Once the medical course of action has been decided upon the parents are likely to gain confidence in their relationships with the infant. The possibility of rejection arises with any abnormal baby, but it should always be remembered that love for a child is very often a slowly developing process. Love at first sight, between a mother and her newborn infant, is probably not a particularly common event. One thing is plain, if the mother refuses to have any contact with the infant no affectionate feelings can develop. Initially her caring behaviour may be rather mechanical, and the relationship vulnerable. It is during that period that a midwife can provide an attentive ear, understanding mind, and an example of accepting behaviour.

WILL PARENTS BE ABLE TO PRE-SELECT THE SEX OF THEIR CHILD IN THE FUTURE?

Recent advances in genetics and fetology bring the possibility of choosing the sex of the offspring somewhat nearer. It is generally assumed, that should parents have the choice open to them more boys would be born. Etzioni (1969) of Columbia University has discussed the social consequences of an effective means of sex selection. As many aspects of social behaviour are sex related, an imbalance in the sexes would have far reaching effects on social life. Women are more average in a number of ways – there are more men at the extremes – intellectually, as subnormal and highly creative and inventive.

There are more male criminals. Women are more conforming and many of them vote conservative in the United Kingdom and Republican in the United States of America. Etzioni claims that American women read more books, see more plays, and generally consume more culture than men. They are also charged with more responsibilities for child rearing and education. All social life is affected by the balance between the sexes. Any large imbalance would certainly reduce the prospect of a well ordered social life. In the United Kingdom a balance between the sexes of marriageable age was achieved during the 1950s for the first time since records started to be kept in 1811. The male habit of going to war periodically, strongly encouraged by the females, successfully reduced each generation of marriageable men. A monogamous society was thus supplied with an excess of young women to provide the labour force in hospitals, schools and the private homes of the more wealthy. The change in the sex ratio has affected these institutions, giving an added force to women's emancipation and altered the attitude of men and women to each other.

REFERENCES

Clare J. E. & Kiser, C. V. (1957) in *Social and Psychological factors affecting fertility*. Ed. Whelpton, P. K. & Kiser, C. V. 5 volumes New York: Millbank Memorial Fund.

Dove, G. A. & Blow, C. (1979) Boy or Girl – Parental choice? *British Medical Journal*, 2 pp 1300–1400.

Etzioni, A. (1969) *Science*, 161 pp 1101–1102.

Hall, M. H. & Carr-Hill, R. (1982) Impact of sex ratio on onset and management of labour. *British Medical Journal*, 285 pp 401–403.

Levine, S. (1961) The psychophysiological effect of early stimulation. In *Roots of Behaviour*, ed. Bliss, E. L. New York: Hoeber.

Mead, M. (1933) *Sex and Temperament in Three primitive societies*. New York: Morrow.

Money, J. (1970) Matched pairs of hermaphrodites: Behavioural biology of sexual differentiation from chromosomes to gender identity. *Engineering and Science* (California Institute of Technology) 33 pp 34–39.

Moss, H. A. (1967) Sex, age and state as determinants of mother-infant interaction. *Merrill Palmer Quarterly*, 13 pp 19–36.

Rosenthal, R. & Jacobson, L. (1966) Teachers' expectancies: determinants of pupils I.Q. gains. *Psychological Reports*, 19 pp 115–118.

Thomas, A., Chess, S., Birch, H., Hertzig, M. E. & Korn, S. (1964) *Behavioural individuality in early childhood*. New York: University Press.

7

Postnatal events

'For the mother, her postnatal care is as important as the birth itself. Unfortunately, in many maternity units it has had the lowest priority, and the mother's joy and satisfaction in the birth of her baby is marred by inadequate and underqualified care, by confusing and conflicting advice and by poor communication between the hospital and the community staff who will care for her and her baby at home' writes Alison Munro, Chairwoman of the Maternity Services Advisory Committee in the Foreword of their Third Report on the Care of Mother & Baby. Chapter 9 on Neonatal abilities is concerned in the main with the baby's needs and activities. These can only take shape and acquire significance in the way they interact with other people – in particular the mother. She too has needs and feelings and may be elated or depressed, contented or agitated, secure or fearful.

In this country mothers are often given their babies to look at, hold, and perhaps to put to the breast when they are born (Fig. 7.1). The infant is usually wrapped in a sheet and this precludes a close examination of him by his mother. By the time mother meets her baby again, he is usually cleanly dressed in shirt and napkin, and warmly tucked under blankets.

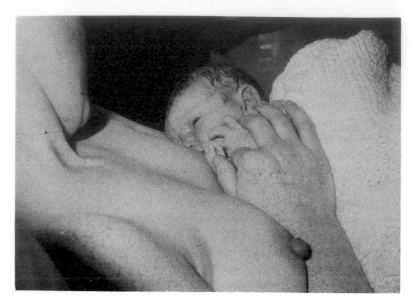

Figure 7.1 Newly born baby at mother's breast.

MOTHER AND BABY'S FIRST CONTACT

Two American pediatricians have filmed a number of mothers with their new babies in their first prolonged contact with them. An overhead heated canopy kept the babies warm so they could be left naked. On analysing the film material, it was found that when mothers are left alone to look at, and examine their naked baby they all follow a similar pattern of behaviour. They touch hands and feet first with their finger tips, and then after several minutes touch his whole body with the palms of the hands. Attempts to get the baby to open his eyes are common and in order to do this they generally support his whole body in an en-face position – that is so that they are face to face, and speak to him. The researchers Klaus and Kennell (1970) have suggested that this sequence of behaviour may be important in establishing early tie of affection between mother and child.

Mothers have complained bitterly that their babies are sometimes whisked away from them after birth, before they have had time to get acquainted. Their need to explore and to get to know their baby is frustrated. Some mothers go home from hospital having never seen their baby naked. A survey done by the Royal College of Midwives (1966) showed that the most common fear of pregnant women is that they will have an abnormal baby. A close inspection has the practical aim of reassurance on this matter; but there is perhaps a less obvious, but very important motivation of making the first steps in an acquaintance process.

SPECIAL CARE UNITS

About 10 per cent of babies now spend some part of the first days of their life in special or intensive care units. In some hospitals parents are strongly encouraged to visit their babies in the nursery. Despite encouragement there are difficulties for mothers in maintaining contact. Harper et al (1976) have found that high levels of contact with babies in special care units, are correlated with high anxiety. Having a very small or ill baby is a worrying event; the special care unit in itself is frightening for many parents (Figs. 7.2a & b). The appearance of the baby is usually very far from the ideal which the mother has been imagining during the months of pregnancy. Not only may her baby's appearance seem bizarre, but his behaviour is quite different from that of a normal baby.

At the birth of a normal healthy baby mothers get very excited when their babies open their eyes. Eye to eye contact has great significance in all social relations. We signal an interest by looking at another person, pay attention to what they are saying by watching their face, and lovers gaze into each others eyes (Fig. 7.3). Traditionally the eyes are the windows of the soul. Small or ill babies open their eyes very little, and it is difficult if not impossible, for their mothers to maintain eye contact with them (Fig. 7.4). In addition, if they cannot handle them they are unable to hold them in an *en face* position.

Bowlby (1969) has suggested that the baby's cry acts to elicit caring and nurturant response in the mother. This sort of behaviour may be less well developed in the mother of a baby whose cry is feeble or infrequent. Moss (1967) has found that mothers pick up their boy babies in the first three months of

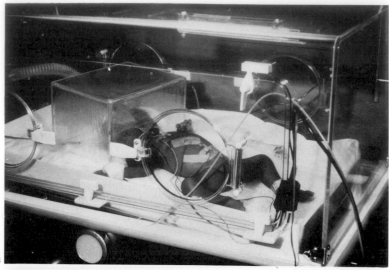

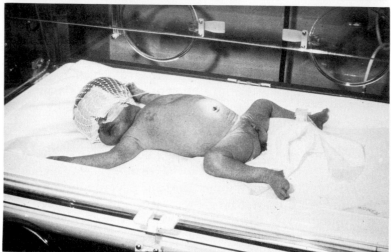

Figure 7.2a & b The need to put babies in special care units can give mothers much anxiety.

life more often than they do girls, and that boys cry more often.

Despite parental anxiety provoked by the birth of a small or ill baby Harper (1976), in the study already mentioned, found that even when the baby died, 90 per cent of parents

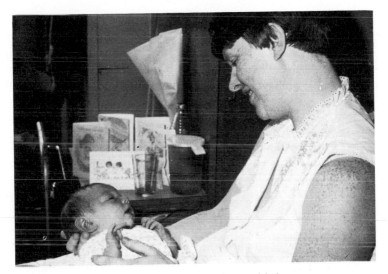

Figure 7.3. Eye-to-eye contact between mother and baby.

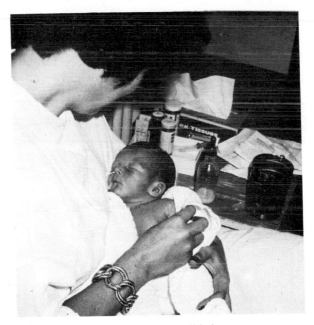

Figure 7.4. Absence of eye contact with an ill baby.

would have opposed any restriction of contact. That is, their motivation to be with their baby is stronger than their motivation to run away from the frightening situation.

Professional staff quickly become familiarised with the apparatus of the special care unit (Fig. 7.5). It can be very chilling to a new mother, who is at the same time having to contend with some rapid hormonal changes within, the worry of a very ill baby, and questioning relatives without. Most special care units are inhumanly quiet, clinically hygenic, and very uncomfortable. The hard metal seats which constitute the furnishings of the units which we know, are hardly designed to encourage prolonged visiting by a mother with perineal stitches.

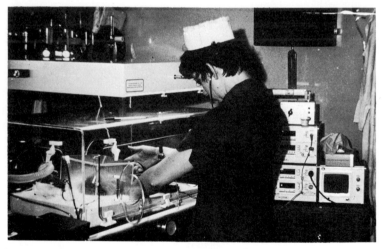

Figure 7.5 Professional staff operating within a special care unit with facility.

The midwife and neonatal nurse have an important job in encouraging the mother to take as much part as she is able, in the care of her baby. The necessary physical care requires a high level of technical competence which most mothers do not have, and there are, therefore problems about role relationships between mother and nurse. A mother can be encouraged to take· an increasing part in helping with the baby's care. Some mothers are initially very frightened to even go near their children, especially those in incubators. A frightened mother who is not supported is likely to visit the nursery less and less. Evidence shows that even with encouragement, the contact between parents and their babies in incubators, is very much less than that between normal babies and their mothers in hospitals (Prince et al 1978). In our experience this can result in the nursing staff becoming critical of the mother and becoming protective and concerned for the baby. By the time the infant is well enough to be transferred to parental care the mother's maternal behaviour may have been seriously disrupted. She may by that time have *got the message* that she is an incompetent mother who cannot manage. The baby who starts life in a special care unit has a somewhat increased risk of being injured by his parents than other healthy children in the same family (Lynch 1975).

Difficulties of pregnancy and delivery which are likely to lead to a baby going to a special or intensive care unit, are more common in the lower socio-economic groups. It is in these socially less favoured families that physically aggressive behaviour is more commonly found. The baby's sojourn in a special care unit is only one of numerous factors which can militate against a good relationship between mother and child. It is therefore of vital importance that the mother become progressively involved with her baby during his stay in the unit.

For the apprehensive mother the rituals associated with entry to a special care unit are daunting (Fig. 7.6). The midwife can be reassuring by accompanying the mother for as long as is necessary, helping her with the procedures for the prevention of infection, and staying with her when she goes to her baby, and encouraging appropriate contact. The father's role is important too. The care of a sick baby is made easier if both parents are involved and there is evidence that support and concern of the father is an important factor in ameliorating a mother's difficulties with her new baby (Blake et al 1975). To witness the passing of a nasal tube on her baby, or to see him have an injection may be very upsetting to a mother. These are procedures which it may be tactful to do in the mother's absence. If they are done when she is present careful explanation should be made beforehand.

The majority of babies born are normal and healthy and some of their mothers are grateful in the first day or two after

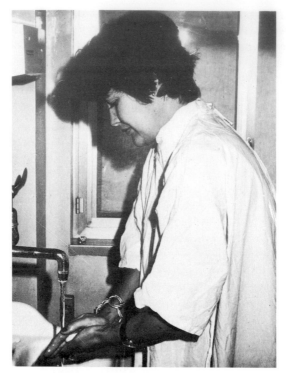

Figure 7.6. Washing hands is just one of the rituals for the mother involved with the special care of her baby.

delivery to be assured of prolonged rest, and are therefore quite pleased if their baby is in a separate nursery at night. Others would prefer to have their babies either in the cot, or in bed with them. One of the advantages of small wards or cubicles is that mothers can have more choice in this matter. It is possible to put three or four mothers who want their babies with them all the time in the same ward. Their infants' sleeping habits will not then inconvenience any mother who wants to sleep soundly all night.

SYNCHRONISATION OF MOTHER AND BABY BEHAVIOUR

It will be clear from the other chapters that many changes take place in the mother after delivery, which enable her to synchronise her activity with that of the baby. In some women the process takes longer than in others. Mothers of first babies have usually had little or no experience of any baby, and the meaning of his signals, how to console, speak to and handle him, all have to be learned. The ease with which this learning is acquired, probably has little to do with intelligence or intellectual achievement. In some respects the highly educated mother may be initially at a disadvantage. Her educational achievements may have required her to develop an analytic style of thinking which can inhibit spontaneous, emotionally responsive, behaviour. It may be a mistake to believe that midwives and pediatricians, for example, with their own first babies, are going to feel good about themselves or their offspring. They may *know* what should be done in an intellectual sense, but experience a delay in the development of the spontaneous inner-sprung need to handle, talk to, be with their baby, which they could describe as loving him. It is rather like learning to ride a bicycle. It is a help to understand about gravity and the principles of balance, but the automatic reactions necessary for smoothly integrated behaviour require additional learning, which comes with practice, and someone who analyses her cycle riding activity minutely may take longer to learn. A midwife should be cautious of assuming that a mother who *knows about* babies can manage her own straight away. She may be the very person who needs more, rather than less, support. She is likely to have more factual information to worry about. 'Is the baby's cord alright . . . has he passed urine . . . are his respirations satisfactory and his airway clear?' The less well informed mother will take it for granted that all the basic functions of her infant are in satisfactory order so she can relax more readily to enjoy his company. In addition, the well informed mother may be reticent in asking advice if she knows the staff expect her to be competent. A midwife, highly regarded by her colleagues professionally, was visited by one of them after she had had her own baby. She looked tired and drawn and the baby was irritable and was said to be losing weight. In the kitchen were twelve assorted tins of milk food! When something goes awry with a highly practised skill, the whole well organised sequence of behaviour can crumble. Panic ensues, and the position can get completely out of control.

Changes in personality and maternal feeling are apparent during the pregnancy. For many women however it is after delivery, when the child they have been waiting for, and thinking about, becomes a reality, that changes in feeling and in role become more noticeable. During the course of a survey of maternal emotional changes, Robson and Kumar studied mothers' reactions to their newborn babies. 40 per cent of primiparae and 25 per cent of multiparae recalled that their predominant emotional reaction when holding their babies for the very first time was indifference. Maternal affection was more likely to be lacking if the mother had had forewater amniotomy, a painful and unpleasant labour or had been given more than 125 mg of pethedine. Most had developed affection for their babies after a week. The postnatally clinically depressed mother was more likely to feel dislike or indifference to her baby at three months. Dana Breen (1975) found in the women with first babies whom she studied that 60 per cent of them thought they had changed since the pregnancy began. Some of the others thought they had changed during the pregnancy, but had reverted to their former selves postnatally. When asked what the most significant aspect of the whole experience of child bearing had been, the most frequently mentioned time was the post-partum period, and relating to the baby. The second most common was the actual birth. This points to childbirth and the postnatal period as being perhaps the critically importance time for personality growth and role modification. The relationship of mother to baby inevitably has an effect on her relationship with her husband, as well as other less centrally placed people (for example the baby's maternal grandmother). Preparatory steps taken in the antenatal period may have provided a *run-in* to the necessary changes but can never completely anticipate them. It is likely that inadequate preparation will mean that some rather abrupt changes will take place at, or fairly soon after, the birth.

ENDOCRINE CHANGES AND MOOD

Most midwives will be familiar with the mild depressive state which afflicts a number of mothers about the third or fourth day after delivery. It is often assumed that *the blues* are normal. In the sense that they occur in a large number of mothers this is undoubtedly true. Yalom et al (1968), for example, found that two-thirds of a group of mothers they studied cried for trivial reasons, realising this was for them unusual. The common cold is in this sense normal, but nevertheless considerable effort is expanded, not only in ameliorating its symptoms, but finding its cause. Little attention is paid to finding the cause of mild postnatal depression, although a number of untested assumptions have been put forward.

Endocrine changes are considerable and affect emotional reactions. It is also on about the third or fourth day that the sudden drop in oestrogen, which accompanies sudden filling of the breasts, is acutely felt. This event may have a more dramatic, though temporary effect on a woman's self-image, than is generally conceded. The breast has become the focus of eroticised sexual interest. Changes in contour and the discomfort of engorged breasts, may arouse considerable sexual as well as maternal anxieties. Women who plan to breast feed often experience two or three days of tearful frustration when the baby finds it difficult to maintain suction. Bottle feeding mothers are increasingly exposed to persuasion to change their minds, and some readily concede that breast feeding is better for their baby. Breast engorgement may, in these circumstances, serve to highlight for them the dissonance between their social-sexual self and their maternal-self.

Within a few days of delivery the majority of women feel physically healthy, and the immediate reason for their being in hospital has passed. Associated with the immediate recovery from delivery may be homesickness and mild depression at being on foreign territory. Women often find they quarrel with one another over small things from about the fourth day. As soon as is possible, siblings should be encouraged to visit (Figs. 7.7a & b). The early transfer of mother and baby home is likely to have a beneficial effect on the family. Other siblings will not be separated from their mother for so long, and the problems that so often follow for the child who is separated from his mother, need not be added to the possibly unavoidable one of jealousy in a

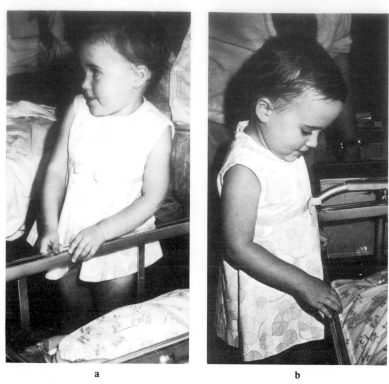

a   b

Figure 7.7a & b Sibling visiting the hospital at the earliest opportunity.

youngster who feels himself displaced. Early discharge is sometimes resisted as being too fatiguing for the mother, especially if there are other young children at home. But one of the symptoms of depression is lassitude, and it may be that effect and cause have been confused. The Dutch, who have a much higher proportion of home deliveries than is currently the case in United Kingdom have a Maternity Home Help Service. Trained home helpers not only assist domestically at the time of the delivery, but help with the running of the household for eight to ten days after the delivery. In the United Kingdom the Home Help service is less specifically trained. A young woman returning home with a baby after 10 days in hospital may face a dispiriting pile of dirty socks, a run-down food cupboard and forgotten rubbish bins. We would speculate that if more effort were expended in helping a woman to maintain her role in relation to other members of the family, and helping her retain control of her own environment the incidence of depression would go down.

Some fathers take annual leave from their work at the time their baby arrives, but paternity leave has not yet been as seriously considered as it should be. The full-time help of fathers for a week or fortnight around the baby's birth may be a factor facilitating early discharge, integrating the family, and giving much needed emotional support to the mother who can then better attend to the new baby. When she is at home she knows it is she who is responsible for the baby's welfare. Inevitably in hospital that responsibility is divided, which is not necessarily to the benefit of normal mothers with healthy babies.

MOTHER'S SLEEP PROBLEMS

Mothers sometimes have sleep problems. These may arise because their babies are night-wakers (see Ch. 6). It may have an endogenous origin in some worry, realistically based or otherwise. A midwife would be well advised to be cautious about a postnatal sleep problem and not to think immediately of hypnotics. The postnatal period requires considerable adjustments to accommodate to a new role, to a new member of the family, to a new family. This cannot always be done overnight and with ease. There may be a lot of worrying to do. 'How will I manage . . . How is my husband going to like it when we both go home . . . How about the other children/my mother/my father . . . How am I going to like it?' As Brenda in *Saturday Night and Sunday Morning* says bitterly to her boyfriend when she discovers she is pregnant: 'What do you think having a kid means? . . . suddenly you're swelling. Then one fine day you're yelling out and you've got a kid. Nowt wrong wi'that. The thing is you've got to look after it every minute for fifteen years. You want to try it sometime' (Sillitoe 1958).

If an opportunity is given to talk about things the midwife may be able to help a mother to think about things in a more constructive way. A few women are genuinely faced with the prospect of losing their husbands because they are jealous of the amount of time their wives spend with the baby. Hypnotics may induce an artificial sleep, create dependence and thereby assure the husband that he was right in thinking that the baby has made his wife neurotic, and the whole thing was a big mistake. A midwife may be able to listen sympathetically to the dilemma of such a patient. It is possible that husband and wife could discuss their problems together with the midwife. She may find she would need to refer the matter to a social worker who has a special understanding of family difficulties.

Many new mothers have no experience of babies and very little relevant information. There are a number of practical matters which may become greatly exaggerated in their minds, and which may not be difficult to set aright. Little things about their baby's appearance, to the midwife quite insignificant, can cause excessive worry. Many mothers, for example, are greatly concerned about forceps' marks on the baby's face, which is extremely unlikely to have anything but a very brief existence. The effects of episiotomy and perineal stitches, abdominal striae and so forth on their sex lives may bother them. Some factual information may be all that is required.

There are other reasons for being cautious about drugs in the puerperium. The over-prescription of drugs, including barbiturates, led to increased use by multiple drug abusers (Ghodse 1976). Prescribing barbiturates is now actively discouraged. Temazepam, a benzodiazepine, is now more popular and, it is hoped, less addictive. In addition, studies of sleep show that there are several different types or stages of sleep, characterised by different patterns of brain activity, and other bodily change, all of which are essential to normal health. A drug-induced sleep has a different pattern from that of natural sleep, and alters the time spent in some stages at the expense of others. On waking, patients rarely feel refreshed as they would from natural sleep. The reason is believed to be that they are suffering deprivation of a particular stage of sleep (Tune 1968).

We have already discussed the effects on their relationship, of either mother or baby being unresponsive. Not only is a mother who is taking hypnotics for sleeping likely to be drowsy, but if she is breast feeding the baby is likely to be somewhat affected.

Mothers are sometimes kept awake by their babies even when they are in hospital. Hospitals vary in the provisions they make for babies at night. Some stay with their mothers, others go to the nursery. The Third Report of the Maternity Services Advisory Committee says unequivocally, 'each mother should normally have her baby at her bedside and take responsibility for his care . . . . The baby should not be moved unless it is at the mother's wish or unless there are overriding medical reasons.' (para 2.2). Some babies are incorrigible night wakers, and the evidence is that it is futile to try to change them. Awkward as it may be for six or nine months, the solution for the mother may be to become a night waker with her infant and to try to organise her life to enable her to do this without too much strain.

It is obvious that sleep and rest which are proper for refreshment and recovery is essential in the puerperium. The effectiveness of drugs in this endeavour is questionable, and brings with it other problems. The measures suggested here might, with benefit, be tried first.

SERIOUS POSTNATAL MENTAL DISTURBANCE

There are more serious and prolonged mental disturbances which can manifest themselves in the postnatal period.

There is disagreement amongst psychiatrists as to the classification of psychoses related to childbearing, but psychoses in the first month after delivery are estimated to occur at the rate of 1 to 2 per 1000 deliveries. A previous mental illness considerably increases the risk of recurrence, and this is far more likely to take place, if it does at all, in the postnatal rather than in the antenatal phase.

Serious depression may result in withdrawal and detachment from the normal day-to-day interest of life. A pervasive black mood descends, making activity seem futile and every event is pessimistically interpreted.

Mania is the other major type of psychotic behaviour. Initially the patient may seem to be unusually ebullient. Jollity, endless activity, and talking continue unabated. The flow of ideas in the speech may become more and more disjointed, and activity destructive.

A schizophrenic episode is marked by disordered thinking, paranoia is not uncommon, and a seeming withdrawal of the patient into herself. Speech may become rambling, and the ideas that are expressed, may seem to have little relationship with one another. The style of the speech also fails to emphasise the emotional importance of its content. In normal speech we draw attention to the main features of our communication by the inflection of the voice; this is often missing in disordered speech.

An acute psychotic episode in the postnatal period may manifest itself by withdrawal and deep depression, paranoia, incongruous emotions and speech, or extreme excitability and activity. In the acute phase the infant is at risk and provision for his protection has to be made. In 1938 the murder of an infant under one year was made a special offence of infanticide, which is dealt with more leniently than murder. The court has to be satisfied that 'the balance of the mother's mind has been disturbed by reason of her not having fully recovered from the effect of giving birth to the child, or by reason of the effect of lactation consequent upon the birth' (Infanticide Act 1938). Giving evidence to the Royal Commission on the Treatment of Mentally Abnormal Offenders, the Governor and Staff of Holloway Prison had this to say:

> Most cases of child murder dealt with by the courts as infanticide are examples of the battered child syndrome in which the assault has had fatal consequences and the child is aged under 12 months. A combination of environmental stress and personality disorder with low frustration tolerance, are the usual aetiological factors in such cases, and the relationship to 'incomplete recovery from the effects of childbirth or lactation' specified in the Infanticide Act is often somewhat remote. (Report of the Committee on Mentally Abnormal Offenders 1975).

This serves to draw attention to situational factors which may contribute to any abnormal behaviour, a very small proportion of which is brought to public notice through the tragic event of a baby being killed by his mother. A few women are proceded against for this offence in England and Wales every year. Such women are at the extreme of those who experience great difficulty in coping with the stresses and strains of life. Part of the stress and strain may well be endogenous but part, as the above extract makes clear, is in the conditions of living with which a woman is faced. These are conditions which can be ameliorated and with which the midwife may be able to help.

The patient will be referred to a psychiatrist and may be removed to a psychiatric unit. Until such specialist help is available the midwife has two important functions. One is to observe the patient's behaviour and make an accurate report about it, and the other is to maintain a high standard of care for mother and baby. The midwife, who is usually not psychiatrically trained, treats the mother with kindness and respect. This is reassuring to other patients who are likely to be alarmed. The common feature of psychotic behaviour is that it is not related to reality. The patient may become extremely agaitated, threatened, or deeply depressed by a remark or an incident which seems unexceptional to anyone else. Abnormal reactions are more often the product of the patient's imagination, however, and she may be deluded or hallucinated. Patients who have recovered from psychotic episodes recall them as extremely frightening and horrifying. It is useless, indeed sometimes dangerous, to try to persuade the patient that she is mistaken in her interpretation of events; it is likely to antagonise her and increase her paranoia. It may be helpful for her subsequent treatment if the midwife can observe whether there is any particular situation, or event, which causes the patient heightened distress. Because she perceives things in an abnormal way her actions are likely to be unpredictable and special care should be taken if she handles her baby. She may refuse to have anything to do with him, or claim that she has never had a baby, or attribute some inappropriate motivation to him. In the interim before she is seen by a psychiatrist, a major objective for the midwife is to *reduce the emotional temperature* and of course to prevent physical harm occurring. The matter will have to be discussed with the husband and possibly other relatives. If the mother is to be transferred to a psychiatric unit, some provision will have to be made for the baby, and this will involve the social worker who can discuss this aspect with the relatives. It is generally agreed that the baby should accompany the mother, and this is arranged wherever suitable facilities exist.

CONTRACEPTIVE ADVICE

The other major concern with which midwives are increasingly faced in the postnatal period is contraception. There have been a number of developments in recent years which are likely to increase the involvement of midwives in family planning. The National Health Service (Family Planning) Act passed on 28th June 1967, enabled Local Authorities in England and Wales to provide a family planning service for all who want it. On 1st January 1975 contraceptive advice and supplies became available under the National Health Service, and on 1st October 1976 Area Health Authorities took over the statutory responsibility for making adequate provision. From 1st January 1976 family planning lectures, tutorials and clinic attendances became part of the midwives training and education, as laid down by the then Central Midwives Board (now the English (Welsh, Scottish or Northen Ireland) National Board for Nursing, Midwifery and Health Visiting).

To some midwives the prospect of becoming involved in the technicalities of fertility control is distasteful. The early birth control clinics in this country were started by people motivated by a desire to see improvements in maternal and child health. It is only since the 1950s and the population *explosion* that the methods used to reduce the burden of large families and improve health and welfare, have been applied in some parts of the world to effect population control policies. The two should not be confused. Family planning involves the free choice and decision of a couple to time the arrival of their children, and to stop having babies when they have enough. They may choose to have none, or two, or twenty-two. Population control may not be possible on the basis of the personal choice of individual couples, as they may choose to have more than is compatible with population control or reduction.

Family planning, to be acceptable and effective, requires the support of other social and health services. In some parts of the world, where population growth is very rapid, attempts to impose limitations on fertility have met with resistance. Many people living in underdeveloped countries still experience a fairly high infant and child mortality rate. Where this is the case, there is a strong motivation to have many children as an insurance for the parents old age, and to safeguard the inheritance of any property there may be. When a family planning service is not associated with maternal and child welfare, and some facilities for the care of the old, then it is likely to be unacceptable. There is a considerable difference for a midwife in being involved in advising couples who want information and guidance on family planning with a view to improving the quality of family life, and being involved in government schemes of population control.

Midwives and nurses may now choose to proceed to a special training course in family planning. Any midwife, however, may be asked for advice about contraception in the post natal period. Many women at that time welcome the opportunity to discuss their own family planning needs and methods, and may be open to influence. The normal procedure is that the earliest family planning consultation takes place after the postnatal examination, and that means six weeks, or perhaps more, after delivery.

A woman with her first baby, may never have organised any method of fertility control before the pregnancy. Some women who have been on the pill need to change their method of contraception for medical reasons. Intrauterine devices have to be re-inserted and cap size may need changing. Altogether a number of patients for a variety of reasons will have no immediate access to contraceptive advice, and no one with whom to discuss the matter for about six weeks.

It is a primary tenet of the family planning service that the only suitable method is that which is acceptable to both the partners. The technically ramshackle method of contraception with which a couple feel content, will be far more effective than the technically perfect system which is for some reason objectionable or distasteful. Large sums of money have been spent on research into inhibiting the biological process of reproduction, but remarkably little attention has so far been paid to the psycho-social factors which are generally acknowledged to be of the utmost importance when a couple come to make a decision about how to limit their fertility. Midwives have a great investment in reducing infant mortality and morbidity, and improving both child and parental health. To be maintained, these improvements have to be associated with effective fertility control.

In this country, between two thirds and three quarters of couples use contraceptive methods which are not doctor related (Wolff 1971, Cartwright 1970). This must surely give us some indication of attitudes to either doctors, or the methods they can make available. There is a variety of contraceptive methods; there are various ways in which these methods may be obtained; and the methods which do exist may require forethought or action by either partner.

Any couple may have attitudes to the method, the means of provision, to each other, or to their own bodies which will affect acceptibility. Positive attitudes of provider and users to each other, and to the method, are necessary if any system is to work efficiently and smoothly. Some of the more technically advanced methods of fertility control are at present only available from a medical practitioner – that is someone specifically trained to deal with illness and disease. At the most vigorous and active stage of life there may be a considerable reluctance to seek advice from a doctor. Doctors are not only associated with illness and invalidity, but also enjoy high status and exercise considerable authority.

There is evidence that potential users of the family planning service desist from doing so because of their dislike of its association with medical formalities (Snowden & Grossmith 1975). Health professionals easily forget what intense foreboding a lay person has at the prospect of being medically examined. In some clinics the medical examination is taken as an opportunity to take a cervical smear. Desirable as this may be from a public health point of view, it is absolutely unrelated to family planning. There is also the very considerable inconvenience of visiting the doctor – often associated with frustrations of waiting. This involves either time off work, finding a baby sitter, or taking the baby along.

The most commonly used methods of contraception are withdrawal and the sheath. The former requires no more than strong will power and the latter access to a slot machine. Withdrawal, in particular, is often not recognised as a method of birth control and is frequently referred to as **being careful**.

It will be apparent that the two methods already mentioned

as being the most popular, are also male methods, although
the sheath should be used in conjunction with a vaginal sper-
micidal pessary to maximise its effectiveness. Couples vary in
their view as to who should take responsibility for their
fertility control. Where the man is the leading partner, then
the likelihood is that he will take effective responsibility in
this matter as in other major matters of concern in the family.
(An IPPF team in Iran dispensed pills to the women – after a
few months only 12 per cent were still adhering to the
scheme. The pills were then dispensed to the men to give to
their wives, 92 per cent were continuing with the programme
months later. In a male-dominated society it was seen to be
important function.) In the context of particular religious or
ethnic minorities – particularly first generation immigrants –
a comprehension of family structure and roles within it is of
major importance if contraceptive advice is to be acceptable.

Some women believe that when they are breast feeding
conception cannot occur, as they do not appreciate that
ovulation occurs prior to the first postnatal mentstrual flow.
This is a misapprehension which the midwife is in a good
position to dispel. She may also need to provide some factual
information about the methods of contraception that are
available, and places in the locality where they can be
obtained.

RETURN TO NORMAL PATTERN OF SEXUAL ACTIVITY

Long-term advice is not often obtained before the
postnatal examination. Abstention for that length of time is
quite impracticable for most couples, who will be strongly
motivated to snuggle down together without too much delay.
There is no period of automatic security against a further
pregnancy following delivery. Withdrawal is associated with
rather high failure rates, so that leaves the condom with
vaginal pessary as the best method to be used until more
detailed family planning advice can be sought.

A patient may be concerned about the effects of perineal
repair or abdominal scarring on the satisfaction of herself and
her husband. Injuries to the pelvic floor which have been
inexpertly repaired may lead to dyspareunia or to dissatisfac-

tions caused by overstretched muscle and connective tissue. Abdominal scars are normally small and neat and are not disfiguring, although both partners may be very conscious of them in the first week or so. Difficulties may be experienced in returning to a normal pattern of sexual activity for psychological reasons. A woman who has had a difficulty pregnancy, labour or delivery, and has been frightened or traumatised by excessive pain, may find her responsiveness dampened.

There is evidence that parents with handicapped children run a higher risk of separating than others. A handicapped child, of course, introduces a variety of strains and stresses into the family. He may, by causing some degree of depression in one or both parents, lower motivation, including sexual motivation. So far as we know, no studies of sexual problems following childbirth have examined this question, though no doubt in the case books of marriage guidance counsellors there is material which could verify or refute the hypothesis.

The human sexual co-ordination of a permanent partnership is a complex affair, involving all aspects of the personality, as well as physical synchrony.

The birth of the baby will change relationships in the family, and possibly occasion some personality development in both parents. The postnatal period is the time of rapid change making considerable demand on a woman's ability to adapt to her new role, new family and new self.

REFERENCES

Blake A., Stewart A, & Turcan D. (1975) CIBA Foundation Symposium 33. *Elsevier Excepta Medica*
Bowlby, J. (1969) *Attachment & Loss: I Attachment*. London: Hogarth Press.
Breen, Dana. (1975) *The Birth of a First Child*. London: Tavistock Publications.
Cartwright, Ann. (1970) *Parents & Family Planning Service*. London: Routledge & Kegan Paul Ltd.
Ghodse, A., Hamid. (1976) Drug problems dealt with by 62 London Casualty Departments. *British Journal of Preventive & Social Medicine*, **30**, No. 4 pp 251–256.
Harper, Rita F., Sia, Conception, Sokal, Sandra, Sokal, Myron. (1976) *Journal of Paediatrics*. **89** No. 3. pp 441–445.
Klaus, H. M. & Kennell, J. H. (1979) Human Maternal Behaviour at first contact with her young. *Paediatrics*, **46** (2) pp 187–192.
Lynch, A. M. (1975) Ill health and child abuse. *Lancet*, **2**, pp 317.

Moss, Howard A. (1967) Sex, age and state as determinents of mother-infant interaction. *Merrill Palmer Quarterly*, **13**. pp 19–36.

Prince, J., Firlej, M. & Harvey, D. (1978) Contact between babies in incubators and their caretakers. In *Early Separation and Special Care Nurseries*, Ed. Brimblecombe, F. S. W., Richards, M. P.M., Robertson N. R. C. London: Heinmann Medical Books.

Report of the Committe on Mentally Abnormal Offenders (1975) Cmnd. 6244. London: HMSO.

Robson, K. M. & Kumar, R. (1980) Delayed onset of Maternal Affection after Childbirth. *British Journal of Psychiatry*, **136** pp 347–353.

Royal College of Midwives (1966) *Preparation for Parenthood*

Sillitoe, Alan. (1958) *Saturday Night & Sunday Morning*. London: W. H. Allen.

Snowden, N. R. & Grossmith, F. J. (1975) Contrasting Trials of use and provision of family planning services. *Journal of Family Planning Doctors* **1**, No. 1, p. 1.

Tune, G. S. (1968) The Human Sleep Debt. *Science Journal*, **4** pp 67–71.

Wolf, Myra. (1971) *Family Intentions*. London: HMSO.

Yalom, I. D., Lumde, D. T., Moss, R. H., Hamburg, D. A. (1968) Post partum Blues Syndrome. *Archives of Genetic Psychiatry*, **18** (1) pp 16–27.

8

Feeding

A number of decisions about the feeding of a new baby have to be made. Is it to be breast or bottle fed? Should feeds be given three hourly, four hourly, or on demand? If bottle feeding is the chosen method, which brand of milk will suit the infant? Who will make up the feeds and give them? To whom will the mother turn for advice, especially when things are not going well. Before reaching her decision she will be influenced in all kinds of ways, both subtle and simple, and the midwife is one of many people who has the opportunity to affect the mother's decision. But it is the mother, ultimately, who must find the answers to these questions in a way which she feels best suits herself and her baby. In some cases where artifical feeding is chosen and is incorrectly prepared there is a risk to the baby of serious complications such as gastroenteritis or hypernatraemia with the risk of brain damage.

There have been fads and fashions in infant feeding throughout history. Only in the 20th century has wider understanding of the biological sciences affected the choice, and in the last decade behavioural scientists have begun to explore some of the factors which affect mother and baby in this central aspect of their early relationship.

HISTORICAL PERSPECTIVE

A review of feeding practices throughout the ages shows how closely they are related to the value put on infant life, and to general social conditions. Babies' feeding bottles have been found by archeologists in parts of ancient Egypt, Greece and the Roman Empire. Some babies were dry nursed, being fed pap or panada. These were mixtures of flour, bread or cereal and milk, or water. One authority writing at the end of the 17th century, complained that such food was 'More suitable for binders to bind their books than for the nourishment of infants', and, indeed, the numerous recipes that were available at that time look very similar to the recipe for flour and water paste! Needless to say, dry feeding was associated with 'summer diarrhoea' contributing to the high mortality rates. But by far the commonest alternative to the mother's breast milk, in cases where the mother was unable or disinclined to feed her own infant, was the wet nurse and this substitute was very widely practised. Some of the earliest wet nurses recorded were slave girls. The peak of popularity of wet nursing in England was reached in the 18th century, and there is little evidence that wet nurses have been much in demand since the mid 19th century. Jane Aitken, however, Chief Midwife to the Nurses' Charity at Guy's Hospital, has this to say in her *Textbook of Midwifery*, the fifth edition of which was published in 1934. 'A wet nurse is the best substitute for mother's milk'. She goes on to list seven essentials which must be sought in selecting a wet nurse. They are that she must be healthy, have firm, full breasts, well shaped nipples, a thriving child of her own a little older than the nursling, a good character, aged between 20 and 30 years, and she must also give up nursing her own child. As the birth rate was very low during the 1930s one can only suppose that there was no great supply of women able and willing to meet these requirements.

Exhortations, usually, but not always, by men, to mothers to breast feed their infants were often realistically accompanied by instructions on the selection of a wet nurse. As in Miss Aitken's *Textbook of Midwifery*, considerable attention was to be paid to the moral character of the woman. There were two reasons for this. The first was the obvious one that parents might have scruples about passing a child to the care of a negligent or malicious woman. The other was based on the strong belief that aspects of the feeder's character, temperament and personality, passed to the child in the breast milk.

ARTIFICIAL FEEDING

Instead of breast milk, the natural sustenance for all mammals for the period immediately after birth, there are reasonable alternatives for human babies. A report of the Department of Health and Social Security in 1974 described the United Kingdom as 'largely an artificially fed', or 'bottle feeding' nation. In 1946, 50 per cent of babies were being breast fed at three months old. The proportion in 1974 was an estimated six per cent. The considerable effort put into persuading and educating that 'Breast is Best' has had results. In the UK in 1980, 88 per cent of babies were being breast fed at 1 week old, 63 per cent at 6 weeks and 40 per cent at four months (OPCS 1982).

Good artificial milk preparations, invaluable for the baby whose mother cannot provide the nourishment, had been indiscriminately recommended, and persuasively advertised. The folly of this has now been widely recognised both in health and social terms.

Some of the disastrous consequences of over-enthusiasm in the use of artifical food are apparent in the underdeveloped countries, where education, hygiene and domestic facilities are inappropriate for the proper preparation and care of artificial food.

Many psychologists have been uneasy for years about the effects of the unnecessary interference with a natural sequence of behaviour that bottle feeding implies. Until recently, however, there has been no evidence of a sufficiently precise nature to provide any influential argument. Evidence from behavioural science more or less coincided with the information implicating artificial feeding of very young babies as a contributory factor in a number of sudden infant deaths. Hypernatraemic dehydration – leading to irreversible brain damage in some cases, and early and severe atopy (allergy) in babies in whose families there is a strong history of eczema, asthma or hay fever, are found more frequently in artificially fed babies than those who are breast fed. This incriminating evidence was that which instigated the Department of Health and Social Security report of 1974, *Present Day Practice in Infant Feeding*, and the memoranda which have followed. *Present Day Practice in Infant Feeding* arose from a concern with the purely physical events (cot deaths, hypernatraemia etc.) the correction of which involves the changing of attitudes, ideas and of established patterns of behaviour, not only for parents but for some doctors, nurses,

Table 8.1 Factors encouraging or discouraging breast feeding

Encouraging	Discouraging
General	
Expert advice favouring breast feeding	Expert advice
Encouragement from other members of the family (mother, husband)	Encouragement from other members of the family to bottle feed
Seeing other mothers breast feeding successfully	Seeing other people bottle feeding
	Advertising of artificial feeding
Early influences	
Breast feeding as seen in paintings and other representational art, by children	
Breast feeding mothers brought into parentcraft and sex education classes in schools, and to antenatal clinics run by midwives and hospitals	
Breast function	
Functional – lactation	Sex symbol – exposure associated with sexual anxiety
Economic efficiency	
Efficiency for mother of a very young baby requires observation responsiveness, patience	Efficiency in many jobs associated with time keeping, speed, precision etc
Education for woman's role	
Maternal role integrated into other roles. Suitable clothing for breast feeding in public, means of baby carrying	Women's liberation movement has concerned itself predominantly with women's role at work, as a sex partner, and socially, and has minimised or denigrated the maternal role

health visitors and midwives. The encouragement of breast feeding advocated by the Department of Health and Social Security report involved a radical change in an important aspect of our culture. In Table 8.1 you will see in diagrammatic form some of the cultural features against, and in favour of, breast feeding.

ATTITUDES TO BREAST FEEDING

Attitudes to breasts and breast feeding are by no means understood and so far little effort has been expended on exploring them. Many attitudes are learned in early life. Children 'pick up' emotional overtones to topics and adopt them as their own. Attitudes to immigrant groups, for example, are affected by parental attitudes. Children imbibe many of the opinions and beliefs of their parents without question. Some recent investigations show that if women believe that they were themselves breast fed they are more likely to do so. In Newcastle 200 newly delivered women were asked to list in order of priority the sources or people who had influenced their choice of feeding method. The results are shown in Table 8.2.

Table 8.2 The sources or people influencing mothers' choice of feeding method (Bacon & Wylie 1976)

| | % of mothers | |
	Breast feeding	Bottle feeding
Their own feelings	95	98
Husband	37	18
Mother	19	18
Hospital	21	7
Friends	20	7.5
Books	18	2
Media	12	2
General practitioner	9	3
Health visitor or midwife	4	1

In a similar study (also in Newcastle) with another 200 women, over half the group had made up their minds about preferred method of feeding before the pregnancy, and only 5.5 per cent decided after the delivery (Eastham et al. 1976).

By far the most important influence is the woman's 'own feelings'. Feelings about particular issues are much the same as attitudes and it is reasonable to suppose that these have been built up as a result of life's experiences. Quite a large proportion of the group located influences in their family (mother and husband). Mothers who chose breast feeding are clearly open to many more influences or, which is more likely, are more of the influences, which affect their judgement. Breast feeding in the United Kingdom is class related. Social class 1 and 2 are not only more likely than Social class 4 and 5 to decide to breast feed, but also are likely to persist for longer (Newson & Newson 1963).

It has been shown that induction of labour and forceps or vacuum deliveries are associated with a delay in starting breast feeding and with higher failure rates (Martin 1978). Palmer et al (1979) found significantly lower breast feeding rates on discharge from hospital to be associated with induction of labour and assisted delivery. The association was unrelated to social class, country of origin, birthweight, anaesthesia in labour or medical reasons for induction or assisted delivery.

KNOWLEDGE OF BREAST FEEDING

The likelihood that a woman having her first baby has had anything to do with a small baby, or has witnessed breast feeding, is remote. For most women their own first child is also their own first experience with a baby. A survey by Jane Hubert in South London published in 1974, showed how deplorably ill-informed a group of working class pregnant women were about conception, pregnancy, childbirth and child rearing. Although they attended the antenatal clinic they were inhibited in asking questions and did not understand much of what went on. From Jane Hubert's report it is clear that much effort put into antenatal education is frustrated by poor understanding. In many antenatal clinics a woman may see a variety of specialists who are likely to examine her with their own particular interests in mind. 'What is the size of the baby's head', 'Should an amniocentesis be done', 'Are there any irregular antibodies' and so on. It must be very difficult for some women to find the right moment and the right person to whom she can put her questions. Having found a midwife willing and able to listen, it may not be easy to frame the questions or express a worry fluently. The midwife, in her role of providing continuity of care has a key task of dealing with the whole person, worries, misunderstandings and all. This may mean translating the technical language and answering straightforward questions. Often, however, the experienced midwife will sense the hidden anxieties and allow the patient to discuss subjects that she feels the doctor may think unimportant.

Acquiring information is one kind of learning; there are others. The baby rhesus monkeys which were brought up with mechanical mother surrogates (see Ch. 1) developed well enough physically. When they grew up, however, their social and sexual behaviour was quite abnormal. They were difficult to mate and those females who did produce offspring had no idea how to look after them. They made cruel, neglectful and murderous mothers. They had had no hand-ling, cuddling, restraining and touching from a parent in their own infancy and it is believed that the absence of this ex-perience prevented them from behaving in a motherly way towards their own babies. It seems likely that human beings learn a lot from being cuddled, picked up and talked to as babies, which they can then pass on to the next generation. It has been found that newly delivered mothers who had been separated from their own mothers experienced more problems with their babies. They also had more marital prob-lems (Frommer 1973).

The study already mentioned in Chapter 1, carried out in Guatamalan hospitals, shows how the contact effected, by putting the baby naked on the mother's abdomen for 45 minutes after birth, and leaving them alone together, affects lactation (Sosa et al. 1976). A follow-up of these mothers and babies shows, amongst other things, that the proportion who are still breast feeding at four months is higher than those treated in the usual way in the hospital. Some writers have suggested that there is a critical period immediately after birth when the mother is especially likely to become attached to her infant. If they are together for that period the mother will become observant and responsive to her baby. If the time passes without the chance of this learning taking place (as may happen if they are separated) there may be difficulties for the mother in accepting the baby happily. The findings from the Guatamalan study suggest that this critical period may have some relevance to the establishment and maintenance of breast feeding. In some parts of the world primigravidae 'borrow' a baby and put it to the breast. This serves not only to prepare the breast antenatally but gives the mother experience in handling and holding a small baby.

The breast is not only a functional organ but also a sex symbol. The cult started in America during the 1920s and the sweater girls of the 1940s ensured that bust size, shape, contour and measurement obtruded into the consciousness of all but the most obtuse. Advertisers lost no time in exploiting the possibilities of sexual anxiety inherent in the characteristics of the bosom. Many young women have become sufficiently dissatisfied with the size and shape of their breasts to undergo plastic surgery, and fear of losing their figure (meaning their breast contour) is a reason sometimes given for refusing to breast feed.

The displacement of sexual interest to the breast has in addition led to potential jealousy sometimes openly expressed by the father of a breast fed baby. Husbands, it will be remembered, were attributed with considerable influence of choice of type of feeding by the sample of women in Newcastle, mentioned earlier in the chapter.

EDUCATION FOR BREAST FEEDING

Midwives, and perhaps more particularly, health visitors, are in a position to influence decisions about health education pamphlets, films, posters and content of talks to schools and mothers. The National Childbirth Trust have some educational programmes in which breast feeding mothers take part. The mother and baby could be presented as a breast feeding relationship in either word or picture. It has been an interesting fact that for years the firms which produce milk feeds for babies, have been at great pains to point out that their product is only second best to the breast! They were quick to appreciate that midwives, health visitors and paediatricians would then look more favourably at their products. The advertisements until recently however showed mothers bottle feeding their very attractive postneonatal babies. One film on breast feeding does present breast feeding, however, almost to the exclusion of the milk product which sponsored its manufacture, and presents it in an attractive and realistic way. It is most helpful for those women who have never seen a baby breast fed.

Better still, antenatal preparation might be helped by the incorporation of one or two mothers who have already had their babies. They could perhaps demonstrate to the apprehensive, the ease with which established breast feeding takes place. Often enough in hospital, the memorable scenes of the early postnatal period when attempts are being made to establish breast feeding are those of some distraught and tearful mothers and hungry frustrated babies. It is not surprising that, with this picture of breast feeding, some abandon the idea and quickly reach for the feeding bottle. If only it were understood that the 'third day problems' and, indeed the whole time in hospital, is quite atypical of the happy relationship which can develop between mother and baby when feeding is properly established. Many mothers and doubtless a few of the younger midwives have probably had no experience whatever of the easy relaxed behaviour which can develop in breast feeding. The third and fourth day problems are rarely discussed in the antenatal period so that breast engorgement and other problems may come as a disagreeable surprise. If potential problems are considered in the antenatal period they may be overcome more readily. No two babies are alike and successful breast feeding will depend on the competence and temperament of the baby being sensitively matched to the competence, temperament and mammary capabilities of the mother. The milk ejection reflex takes some days or weeks to get established. A mother can be reassured of this very early on. Perhaps one of the more powerful and beneficial influences in a hospital ward is an experienced mother. Experimental studies of small groups demonstrate clearly the existence of 'informational social pressure' that is, in conditions where members of a group are unsure about what to do, an individual with relevant experience wields influence. A few breast feeding multiparae, well placed, could be a valuable resource to any midwife trying to encourage breast feeding.

Such mothers may also be able to demonstrate the fact that there is little direct relationship between breast size and milk supply. It is often claimed by the uninformed that the possession of small breasts rules out the possibility of breast feeding and pregnant women often express their anxiety about this. There are a few studies reported of mothers' attitudes to breast feeding but none concerning those of the people who are likely to attend her. The Association for the Improvement of the Maternity Services has found that mothers complain that one of the difficulties in establishing breast feeding is that they get inadequate or conflicting advice. This is not surprising as the most experienced midwives spend much of their time in administration and in initiating into ward policy and routine student midwives and obstetric nurses, some of whom stay for only a few weeks. Some units do the same with medical students and others grades of learners. The patients have, therefore, most contact with the least experienced staff who are not in a position to give suitable answers, but feel they must say something! More permanent members of the ward team are often part time which adds to the variety of advice and views, not all of which are up to date.

It seems often to be assumed that midwives themselves are all, by nature, not only in favour of babies being breast fed, but competent and at ease in discussing breast function and in giving practical aid and advice. Midwives, no less than their patients, are subject to the cultural influences which bear upon them. Personal feelings and professional tasks often need to be kept apart; experienced midwives and health visitors have probably evolved ways of doing this. But there may be a case for providing students with some facility for discussing conflicts and 'hang-ups' they may have about breasts and breast feeding.

DIFFICULTIES CREATED FOR BREAST FEEDING IN HOSPITAL

People who are required to implement a policy to which they feel antagonistic, consciously or otherwise, are unlikely to be successful. Many mothers find breast feeding is much easier once they get home on their own territory. There are many aspects of hospital life which interfere with smooth relationships between members of a family and this is particularly so with a new member. During the later weeks of pregnancy some sort of 'nest building' activity is often apparent. Preparing a room, buying clothes and paraphernalia, delineating the territory, is part of preparatory behaviour. At the very moment of zero hour the mother is transferred to alien territory where, in the medicalised setting, she takes on some aspects of the 'sick role'. The more thorough the medical attention she receives the more this role is enforced. Part of the sick role is to transfer responsibility. From the patients' point of view, at some times of the day a ward can look like a railway station in the rush hour, with everyone seemingly bent upon his (or her) own business. Staff, trained, or learners of varying abilities, appear unexpectedly to either help with feeding or gather information. Doctors may do a rapid ward round between clinics or labour ward work. In addition to ward staff there may be physiotherapists, laboratory staff, research workers and a variety of paramedical and social work personnel. In pursuit of their own tasks they inevi-

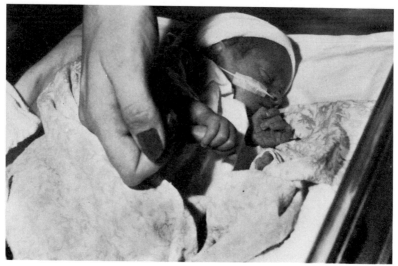

Figure 8.1 Baby grasping mother's fingers.

tably interfere with individuals and can seriously disturb a mother whose baby is not yet feeding satisfactorily.

Even with early discharge home some of the most important experiences for mother and baby will have passed in hospital. At birth a normal full term baby has a number of reflexes present, which can be thought of as a rudimentary survival kit. The grasp, plantar, rooting and sucking reflex enable him in an emergency to hold on to mother and suck. These reflexes gradually give place to more discriminating learned behaviour. An older infant has learned what sort of objects bring a reward. There are, however, two kinds of sucking – nutritive and non-nutritive. Anyone who has watched small babies will have seen that they spend some time of each day 'mouthing' (i.e. moving their lips as if sucking). They also suck their fingers or a piece of blanket. Most young mammals engage in some non-nutritive sucking which is not necessarily related to hunger. Puppies who are given large feeds in a short time do a lot of non-nutritive sucking, as if they needed to perform a certain amount of activity. Breast fed babies do more non-nutritive sucking than bottle fed babies (Richards & Bernal 1972). Indeed the whole pattern of sucking, breathing and swallowing is different in bottle fed than in breast fed babies. Non-nutritive sucking is often looked upon as an index of alertness, and is usually seen very soon after birth. Within a few minutes of being born some infants are vigorously sucking their fingers, yet it may be several hours before they are put to the breast. All newborn mammals make strenuous efforts to find the nipple. A healthy newborn baby held near to the breast will, by the functioning of the rooting reflex, find the nipple (though he is usually helped in this). From the moment he is born, learning about the environment takes place very rapidly. A baby who is put to the breast very shortly after birth possibly has this as his first positive learning experience. He will be learning about the shape and texture of the nipple, the smells, sounds and feelings (kinesthetic experience) that go with it. Babies will suck on a nipple or teat even when no food is forthcoming, while they remain unresponsive to food provided by a spoon. The experience of drawing the nipple to the back of the mouth seems to act as an initial reward in itself, and this is subsequently reinforced by the flow of milk. Two points follow: one is that the sucking is a good experience on its own. The fact that a small but nutritive amount of colostrum is the only food reward is not important. The other point is that the early learning about the smell, sounds, textures and so on, that are associated with feeding are very special: they may be the first learning that the baby does and they are very individual. Every mother has a particular smell, voice, way of holding her baby, and these characteristics are associated with feeding. The gradual development of a positive response to the breast may easily be disturbed in the early days by someone else giving a complementary feed. The satisfaction of hunger is particularly likely to be associated with a lot of incidental learning so if we want the baby to learn how to breast feed it is better not to provide alternative learning situations for him. There is considerable

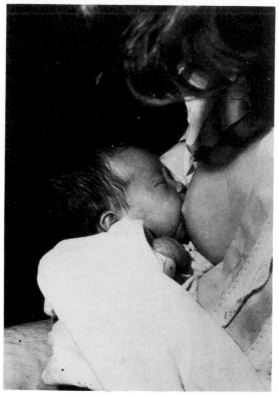

Figure 8.2 Baby breast feeding.

evidence that mothers who are left on their own with their babies and encouraged to feed them on demand find it easier to establish breast feeding than in the cases where the care of the baby is divided in the first few days between nurse and mother.

On the mother's side her mothering role is likely to become stronger when she is left to work things out on her own. She may need some encouragement or even some suggestions as to how she might proceed in order to build her self-confidence. This is particularly important in a nervous patient who wishes to have a specified routine round which to organise her life, especially where family influence with regard to fixed interval feeding, has been strong. It is sometimes extremely difficult in a hospital setting to avoid undermining maternal confidence. The boundary between advising and interfering is usually somewhat fragile. There is the added difficulty in a hospital that the complexity of the apparatus, the efficiency and speed of the staff working under various constraints, the mechanisation, all manage to convey the impression that having and caring for a baby is a highly technical affair, only to be understood after years of experience or specialised training. During labour both mother and fetus are apt to become entangled in machinery incomprehensible to all laymen who are not electronically minded. After the baby is born it may need specialised attention. The likelihood is that it will be found whole and healthy, not by the inspecting eye of its own mother but by a highly trained midwife or paediatrician. An enquiry conducted by the National Childbirth Trust brought many complaints from mothers that after the birth they did not see their baby for some hours. The provision of a high level of specialised physical care can give the patient the impression that she is somewhat inadequate to care for her baby. There are probably few mothers, especially mothers of first babies, who do not feel they should take a subordinate role while in hospital. The hospital is alien territory – patients are there as guests and no guest feels it proper to be dominant in his host's home. A breast feeding relationship, however, is a primary and central one which is easily disrupted in hospital.

Because of the 'emergency' nature of a lot of hospital work and the demands of many and varied learners, hospital trained staff not infrequently have to develop a directive style of leadership. While suitable, indeed necessary, in many situations which arise in a hospital, it is not always helpful to a woman vacillating about her choice of feeding method. Attitudes to breasts and breast feeding are the products of life long subtle influences, and have strong emotional overtones. Emotional responses are rarely changed by direct factual information. In the Newcastle survey, already referred to, a third of the bottle-feeding mothers agreed it would be better for their baby to be breast fed. This knowledge did not however override their antagonistic feelings. There is quite a lot of evidence that if people are given unwelcome advice they are likely to strengthen their already existing attitudes. Their opinions may then move further away from that being advocated and also lead to a rejection of the source of the information as well, as the Newsons' study (1963) in Nottingham showed. There, some mothers rejected not only the advice but the health visitor herself together with the whole profession. This is a result entirely predictable where information, or instruction is given to an antagonistic audience. A more realistic attempt might be made if attitudes to breasts, breast feeding, having babies and rearing them could be brought out in an openended, non-directional discussion in a one-to-one or group setting. Cryptic leadership in such situations is a skilled task requiring not only the ability to listen and *hear*, but also to be able to tolerate and, if necessary, share the anxieties, aggressive feelings and other strong emotions that may be expressed.

COMPOSITION OF BREAST MILK: EFFECT ON FEEDING PATTERN

As was mentioned in the Introduction, human breast milk is dilute and close in composition to the milk of other mammals who are continuous feeders. The study of a wide range of mammals shows that feeding patterns are intimately related to milk strength. Mammals with highly concentrated milk may feed their young as infrequently as once in 24 hours, while others with dilute milk carry and feed their offspring more or less continuously. The interval between feeds of different mammals has been found to be related not only to milk composition and growth rate of the young but also with the style of infant care (Ben Shaul 1962). Some mammals make nests where the young are left for long periods (e.g. rabbits), others, like most monkeys, carry their offspring, who are able to cling on. The infants of most cloven footed mammals follow the mother from almost immediately after birth. The opportunities for feeding with these different kinds of infant care vary. It is now clear that in species which have concentrated milk there are long intervals between feeds, short feeds, and a high rate of sucking by the offspring. Conversely, dilute milk is associated with the reverse pattern. The details of this are less important than the general notion that a whole range of different factors are interdependent. A change in one of the factors may disrupt the smooth sequence of important activity.

Most of the artificial feeds available for babies are more concentrated than is human breast milk and this change may disrupt the natural pattern of sleeping, sucking and other activity of the infant. A group of breast fed and artificially fed babies were carefully monitored at Birmingham Maternity Hospital. All were fed four hourly for six feeds a day. The average intake and weight gain of the breast fed group was significantly less than the artificially fed. Early and more frequent feeding is essential if the mother who desires to breast feed is to be encouraged by practical success (Culley et al 1979). There are marked periodicities in normal infant feeding – the baby sucks quite vigorously for some seconds, rests, and then returns to sucking until another rest period. Breast and bottle fed babies have quite different patterns of sucking and resting resting. Not only do the babies behave differently but breast-feeding mothers, it has been found, interact with their babies between the bouts of sucking. It is then, during the rest period, that they may look, or smile, or talk to their babies. Bottle-feeding mothers are less phased in with their infants' activity in this way. A study in Cambridge in which mothers kept detailed diaries giving details of their daily activities, showed that successful breast-feeding mothers fed their babies more often. The mothers were found to be more responsive to their babies' needs and less constrained by preconceived ideas about what ought to be done. It was clear from that study that four hourly feeds are too infrequent for some babies and that, particularly when the night feed is omitted, a rigid adherence to the clock may result in the infant being underfed. An essential feature of successful breast feeding is a relaxed relationship in which the mother can respond to her baby and learn from her observation of him. Babies, we now know can see much more than was previously believed. For them the mother is not just food but has a particular face to be looked at and explored, and a particular way of holding to be enjoyed and so on. Most mothers need an enhancement of their self-confidence, so that they can be satisfied with what they are doing in the vital steps in making a relationship with their baby. A good relationship cannot be built from a set of instructional rules. Observation and responsiveness are two essential ingredients and it is in these kinds of activity that mothers can be encouraged. Some may need rather more practical guidance than others. New babies can look very fragile and untouchable to someone with no previous experience of them. A simple word suggesting that a mother pick up her crying baby may still be necessary initially. Newly delivered mothers do not, generally speaking, have a reputation for high intelligence amongst the staff. To be uncertain about how to proceed can be guaranteed to make *anyone* seem foolish. Were she in her own home much of the new mother's uncertainty would be resolved. The midwife has the vital task of helping a mother to resolve her uncertainties about the way she handles her baby, and as far as possible, to resolve many of the uncertainties intrinsic to the hospital situation. This may require suggestions and encouragement but not direct interference.

One of the disappointing features of the smaller four or six bedded wards is that the midwife cannot be so observant and her visits to the ward must usually seem more intentional. The older type of large ward, with its many disadvantages, at least provides an opportunity for unobtrusive observation or suggestion. Babies differ widely in all kinds of ways, the amount and timing of their sleep and wakefulness, their alertness, crying and speed with which they adapt to noise and other stimuli. We will discuss individual differences of babies in more detail in Chapter 10. The point here is that some of the characteristics of a baby (for example the timing of his sleep) persist for months, sometimes years. As there are such wide variations from child to child a set of rules is likely to be inappropriate for some children. The responsiveness and flexibility required of a new mother is behaviour which most of us have been carefully trained *not* to do. The ideal of efficiency so pervasive in any advanced society, means going to school on time, catching trains, being at work – doing things by the clock. Innumerable psychological studies documenting differences between the sexes find men to be more task orientated, ambitious, assertive and women more person orientated, and affiliative.

BREAST FEEDING AND THE WORKING MOTHER

The changes in the role of women have been most apparent in the work setting. Almost all jobs are now in theory open to both men and women. Equality in the sex partnership and in the social role has also been largely achieved. Women with, or wanting babies, have been ill catered for by the various moves for the emancipation of women. The mother's role, if it is not to impose undue strain on some women, or indeed some families, needs to be more fully integrated into other roles that modern women occupy. As much of our economic and social lives is conducted outside our homes, child-rearing unavoidably adds a dimension to living which requires energy and planning if it is to be coordinated with an economic and social life. The traditional view that this makes a dual-role demand on women is giving place to the more egalitarian idea that it makes demands of both parents. Indeed, it is the shared parenting ideal which has often made bottle feeding attractive. The evidence against early bottle-feeding, however, requires some modification in the provisions for the post-partum period.

Some of the traditional women's costumes of Europe and Asia were functional in this respect and it is easy to see how breast feeding could take place without any public exposure. In the last decade there have been great improvements in facilities available so that a baby can be carried on the body (see Fig. 8.3). This form of baby transport by maintaining

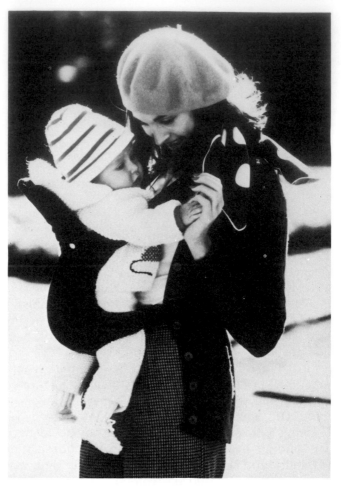

Figure 8.3 The sling is one way of conveying a baby without the mother needing to hold it. (Photograph by courtesy of Little Rock Ltd.)

close proximity of mother and baby encourages a relaxed relationship which is integral to breast feeding. The grand perambulators which accompanied nannies on their course through life have largely given place to lighter more adaptable prams which can be put into cars and buses, which again helps the easy acceptance of the baby into family and social life.

In parts of the world where babies are carried and suckled on demand a crying baby is hardly ever heard. Resistance to admitting babies to public places and to some working situations would possibly be less if this were an accepted pattern of behaviour. There are some jobs which could be made compatible with the care of a small baby. A teacher, midwife or health visitor with an accompanying breast-fed baby would provide a very good practical example and many hospitals now provide a crèche for their staff.

Many women feel extremely tired a few weeks post-partum. There are two psychological situations which can be guaranteed to make the most vigorous feel exhausted. One is boredom and the other is to be indecisive over a personal conflict. The tiredness is usually explained physiologically. It may equally be accounted for psychologically. The smelling salts and vapours which were all accepted as part of the life for the constrained, frustrated Victorian middle class women were in part caused by the rigours of enclosing corsetry and in part by the utter boredom and ennui of their respectable lives. Much less is heard of the 'vapours' since the *ennui* has been dispelled. *Ennui* is a mental weariness stemming from lack of occupation or interest. It characterised the lives of Victorian women, and at one time its high incidence in convents was of great concern to the church. Many of our assumptions about women with very young babies are that they will stay at home, foregoing many of their interests. What situation could be better calculated to induce conflict and boredom? There is much that could be done, and midwives and health visitors are in positions where they can often initiate or influence decisions for improvements.

To summarise: the smooth integration of a new baby into the family would be facilitated if the mother were able to continue in some of her previous activities, if not all. To an unnecessary extent the arrival of a new baby, especially the firstborn, often requires the mother to alter her life in a restrictive direction. Changes in women's social and work roles, have not yet fully accommodated the mothering requirements. There are many indications that these are being neglected or relegated to a secondary position with great cost to society.

REFERENCES

Bacon, C. J. & Wylie, J. M. (1976) British Medical Journal, 1 pp 308–9.
Ben Shaul, D. M. (1962) The composition of the milk of wild animals International Zoological Year Book, 4 pp 300–332.
Culley, P., Milan, P., Roginski, C., Waterhouse, J. & Wood, B (1979) British Medical Journal, 2 pp 891–893.
de Sweit, M., Fayers, P., Cooper, L. (1977) Lancet, 1 pp 892.
Department of Health and Social Security (1974) Present day practice in infant feeding.
Eastham, E., Smith, D., Poole, D. & Neligan, G. (1976) British Medical Journal, 1 pp 305–307.
Frommer, E. A. (1973) British Journal of Psychiatry, 123 p 573.
Hubert, J. (1974) Belief and reality: social factors in pregnancy and childbirth. In The Integration of the child into the Social World, Ed. Richards, Martin P. M. London: Cambridge University Press.
Mackintosh, J. M. (1947) British Medical Bulletin, 5 pp 185–7.
Martin, J. (1978) Infant Feeding 1975. London: HMSO.
Neville, J. (1976) The Times 7th April.
Newson, J.& Newson, E. (1963) Infant care in an urban community. London: Allen & Unwin.
O.P.C.S. (1982) Infant Feeding. Martin, J. Monk,
Palmer, S. R.,Avery, A. & Taylor, R. (1979) The influence of obstetric procedures and social and cultural factors on breast feeding rates at discharge from hospital. Journal of Epidemiology & Community Health, 33 pp 248–252.
Richards, M. P.M., & Bernal, J. F. (1972) An observational study of mother-infant interaction. In Ethological studies of child behaviour, Ed. Blurton-Jones, N. London: Cambridge University Press.
Sosa, R., Kennell, J. H., Klaus, M. & Urrutia, J. J. (1976) The effect of early mother-infant contact on breast feeding, infection, and growth. In Breast Feeding and the Mother, Symposium 45. London: CIBA Foundation.

9

Neonatal abilities

Frederick Leboyer in his *Birth Without Violence* (1974) asks why nobody is concerned about the sufferings of the baby during birth. Considerable atempts have, after all, been made to relieve the pains of the mother for over a century. The answer he suggests is in the very commonly held view that new babies have no conscious awareness, that they can neither hear nor see and are incapable of intense feelings. William James who was appointed to the first ever Professorship in psychology in the 1890s described the world of the newborn as he imagined it, in the following terms: 'The baby assailed by eyes, ears, nose, skin and entrails at once feels that all is one great blooming buzzing confusion' (James 1890). He seems to have thought that babies were capable of seeing and hearing, but that they were unable to organise the experience or to make any sense of it. This has been a commonly held view until recently. Some of the older textbooks on baby care and child development, go so far as to claim that a newborn infant is unable to see.

Many people who have a lot to do with new babies, have often wondered whether the experts are right. In the main we judge how a person experiences the world, by what he does or what he tells us about it. A new baby can do little of either, so it has been assumed that he experiences little. A similar

139

idea sometimes prevails with a patient who seems to be unconscious, partly conscious, or has had a stroke. He can neither speak nor move; conversations take place over him, and discussions about him, which assume that he is deaf to the world, and without understanding or memory. Sadly this is often not true. He may be doubly distressed: first by what he hears, and secondly by his inability to make this fact apparent to anyone. This is an experience incidentally, which occasionally occurs during a light anaesthetic, preceding the delivery of the baby in a caesarean section.

SENSORY AND PERCEPTUAL ABILITIES OF THE NEONATE

In trying to find out more precisely how newborn babies experience the world about them, a number of experimental techniques have been developed in the past few years, which have shown that despite his restricted motor capabilities, the human neonate has sensory and perceptual capabilities far beyond those accorded him. The techniques used in *asking* a newborn baby what he can perceive, what he prefers and remembers, depend on the measurement of motor activity (head turning, visual fixation, sucking etc.) and on physio-logical measures, for example, cardiac and respiratory changes, galvanic skin response and electro-encephalo-graphic changes. A stimulus may evoke a particular activity or it may stop an activity. Some of these responses may be apparent to any careful observer. An example of this being that a particular sound may induce a baby to change his facial expression, or to disturb him from a restful state. If he is feeding, the same sound may cause him to stop sucking. These ways of responding are common enough to all of us. We turn with a *what's that?* expression to a new or unusual sound. If we happen to be doing something demanding our close attention, we stop to give full attention to the new stimulus. The orienting response and the cessation of other behaviour are both signs of being alert. When alert, both baby and adult are more perceptive. Alertness can be thought of as an increase in the general level of functioning. It is usually followed by organised attention to a particular feature of the environment, and the mobilisation of resources to deal with the stimulus. Recall, for example, a baby aroused for feeding. He becomes more active and bright, his activity then narrows down and becomes concentrated on the nipple and sucking, so that we can see the sequence: alerting, attention, action.

The techniques which have been used to assess perceptions and preferences of the newborn, depend on the careful observation and recording of motor activity and physiological changes. Using these techniques it is clear that neonates do perceive a great deal that was previously thought to be beyond their comprehension. Two other commonly held views of newborn babies may also have to be changed in the light of evidence. The first is that activities of a new baby occur only in response to stimuli, either from outside or from internal organs. This concept has to give place to that of an active little creature, who initiates things himself, and affects the behaviour of his parents, as well as responding to what happens to him. Secondly, a fairly commonly held idea, that babies are all alike and develop individuality as a result of their experiences will have to be modified to acknowledge a wide range of individual differences present from birth.

The picture which emerges of the newborn is that he has a considerable ability for perceiving his surroundings and for selecting some aspects as being more interesting and worthy of more prolonged attention. Secondly, he can initiate a sequence of behaviour as well as responding to outside stimuli. From the beginning of life he may show quite individual qualities of temperament, emotional traits and character which will contribute to his adult personality.

Long before he can explore his surroundings by direct touch, or by crawling and walking, he can explore with his eyes. Robert Fantz, a psychologist at Western Reserve University, U.S.A. has found that babies of a week old show a distinct preference for complex rather than simple visual patterns (Fantz 1961). The baby, lying supine in the cot, had a series of pairs of patterns on the *ceiling* of the viewing box placed over the cot, at which he could look. A small peep hole in the ceiling and appropriate illumination enabled the experimenter to see the images of the pattern on the ceiling mirrored in the baby's eyes. When the baby looked directly at one of the patterns, the image over the pupil could be seen by the experimenter. The experimenter then recorded the amount of attention given to each pattern. The results show clearly that the more complex pattern receives more attention. For example, a red and white chequer board pattern has more than twice the attention of a plain red square of the same size alongside it. The pattern which has by far the most attention is that of a human face. The neonate looks most intently at an object which is at a distance of about 9 or 10 inches (23 to 25 cm) away from his eyes. The mammary glands being between the 2nd and 6th rib, ensures that when breast feeding the mother's face is just about that distance from the baby. She is positioned, therefore, for maximum learning if she looks at her baby in an *en face* position. It has been found, however, that a larger number of breast feeders closed their eyes while feeding, and that when they do open their eyes, they do not necessarily look at the mother's face, but at the breast tissue (Infant Feeding Project, Wright, Crow and Fawcett, Edinburgh University). Some bottle feeding positions can extend beyond the optimal visual range of the infant. In a further development of this experimental technique, it has been shown how a newborn baby scans a pattern by visual exploration (Salapatek & Kessan 1966). Pictures are taken which record the movements of the infant's eyes. When presented with a triangle the babies concentrate on the angles, so that the scanning pattern looks like this diagram (Fig. 9.1).

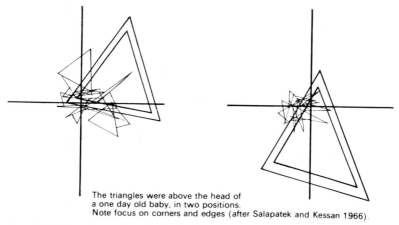

The triangles were above the head of
a one day old baby, in two positions.
Note focus on corners and edges (after Salapatek and Kessan 1966).

Figure 9.1 Visual scanning of triangles by the newborn.

This work shows clearly that a newborn infant does explore visually, and that some features of the environment do attract more attention than others. The *human face* pattern possibly has some important evolutionary significance. It is perhaps of elementary importance that the young should be able to distinguish adults of their own species without delay. These experiments, however, help us to describe what the infant does, rather than why he does it. He explores visually; particular objects attract his attention; he can focus on them and scan them.

A much earlier study (Chase 1937) showed clearly that babies of 15 days old could discriminate among a range of colours. In studying colour discrimination, however, it is not clear whether the infant is responding to brightness or to hue. Yellow, for example, is brighter than blue and is also a different hue. Hue, which is the dimension of blueness or yellowness, depends on the wavelength of the light, and brightness on the amplitude of the wave. It is not clear either, whether babies of under 16 days can distinguish between one colour and another.

In view of the neonates locomotor helplessness, vision is a most important avenue for learning, and getting to know

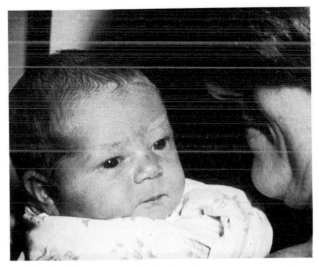

Figure 9.2 Baby looking over mother's shoulder becomes visually alert.

the world he lives in. It will be a common enough experience to midwives that when babies are picked up to be consoled, they are often held so that they are looking over the adult's shoulder (Fig. 9.2). When this happens many babies stop crying and become visually alert. Opening the eyes in this way does not happen when the infant is simply handled, nor when he is placed in an upright position only (Korna & Grobstein 1966). The opportunity to look round and to experience the world may play a crucial role in early development. A mother who holds her baby in an upright viewing position is inadvertently also providing him with new experiences, and an opportunity for learning. Much attention has been paid to the influence of maternal care and handling on the development of emotional security. It is also proper to consider the effect of maternal behaviour on the intellectual development of the infant. When a mother picks up her baby, she is aiding both the development of emotional security by providing warmth and assurance and at the same time, widening his perceptual field, and thereby encouraging his intellectual development.

PREFERENCE FOR MOTHER'S FACE

Mention has already been made of the preference neonates show for a black and white model of a human face, over a patterned stimulus. Genevieve Carpenter (Carpenter et al, 1970) found that from the age of one week, a baby responds differently to his mother's face and that of a model. It can be inferred therefore, that some recognition of the mother's face is possible. Recognition is only possible if something is remembered. The idea that a baby can remember anything at a week old, would probably not be conceded by most people working with mothers and young babies on the basis of normal observations, and shows both the value and the need for, special techniques for observing and recording infant behaviour.

If babies are able to both perceive and learn, at such an early age, fresh questions arise about their care in hospital, in the immediate post-natal period. We have already seen in the Chapter on Feeding (see Ch. 8) that breast feeding is prolonged when mother and baby are in close proximity for about an hour after birth. It has been assumed that the mother is favourably influenced by the opportunity to inspect and handle her new baby without interference. We now have to consider the effect on the baby of a prolonged opportunity of examining his mother's face. Mother and baby's inspection of each other provides the opportunity for each to learn about the other (Fig. 9.3). In adulthood mutual gaze has always been recognised as an important means of communication. The eyes have been referred to romantically as the *windows of the soul* and prolonged eye-to-eye contact is traditionally associated with falling in love. The mother may never again have the freedom to spend such long periods of time looking at, cuddling, and nursing her baby. Mothers often become quite excited if their babies look at them. The care and attention the mother gives her baby is made much more rewarding by an attentive infant. The potential opportunities for mother and baby should be recognised and given due weight in considering all the practical requirements which may lead to interfering between mother and baby and disrupting their relationship.

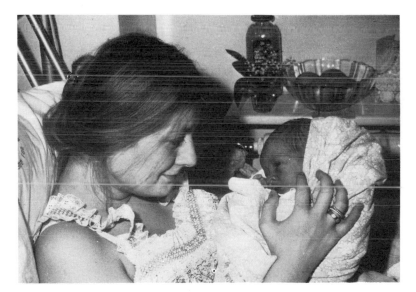

Figure 9.3 Mother and baby inspecting each other at the earliest opportunity.

VISUAL ABILITIES

Greenman (1963) has found that 95 per cent of normal infants, normally delivered, can follow an object visually. He used a four inch (10 cm) red ring at approximately 10 inches (25 cm) from the face, when the baby was supine, within 96 hours of birth. Where central nervous system damage has occurred the moro reflex, grasping, automatic walking are usually normal, but it is the visual following which is lacking. This may clearly affect the social relations between mother and baby. A moderate degree of photophobia during the first few days of life has been noted. The study of the visual behaviour of newborn babies usually has to be done in a subdued light, or the infant will not open his eyes at all. It has also been found that babies not only look round in the dark, but they open their eyes and actively *search* by scanning when the light is put off (Haith 1972).

Reduced illumination is one of the features of Leboyer's method of delivery, and favourable comment has been made about the apparent alertness of the infants, which may, of course, be due to other features of his method. Whether an infant's eyes are open or shut is likely to affect both his social relations and his learning. In normally sighted human beings the very great majority of information about the world comes through the eyes. There are important things to be learned in the first few days of life, and this is the time when social communication between mother and baby begins.

The ability of the very young of several species of animal to perceive depth, has been established by the use of a test apparatus known as a visual cliff (Gibson & Walk 1960). This consists of a patterned chequered floor with a raised platform of the same pattern. The platform is covered with a glass plate which extends right over the lower section. Young animals placed on the platform side will explore, but always stop at the platform edge. The *drop* is visible, although the glass plate provides a continuous firm flat floor. Young children who can crawl have been tested with the visual cliff, and they too stop at the cliff edge (Fig. 9.4).

A crawling baby has several months in which to learn about depth, however, and this tells us nothing about the neonate. By comparing recordings of the heart rate of very much

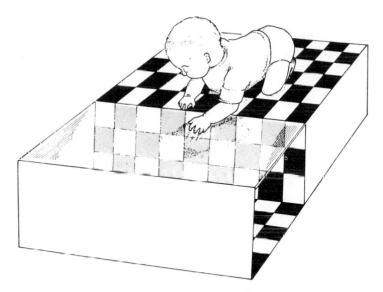

Figure 9.4 Child stops at the visual cliff edge of a patterned platform (after Gibson and Walk).

younger babies placed over the shallow and the deep side it is plain that they can discriminate the difference. Neonates have not been tested in this way yet, but what does emerge is that babies of eight weeks old show no distress outwardly but a marked response of their autonomic system. Older children show marked distress. It has been suggested (Campos, Langer & Krow 1970) that there is a developmental delay between the ability to distinguish a stimulus, and the ability to communicate the fact by an emotional response. The limitations of their emotional expression may not reflect limitations of their experience. In other words, it is unjustified to assume that because a new baby fails to smile, he is not experiencing pleasure, or because he does not show boredom he is not needing something interesting to look at or listen to. The experience which is accumulating in the early days and weeks will be of the greatest importance at a later stage. With increasing physical maturation he will be able to act on information acquired earlier.

Jean Liedloff (1975) mentions an incident in which an American child who was prevented by fences and locked gates from exploring in the family swimming pool area. When it finally got through the barricade it fell in the pool and was drowned. She contrasts the behaviour of parents and child in this setting with that of the Yequana, a primitive jungle tribe of Venezuela, with whom she had spent two and a half years. Children there play unsupervised around a pit and never get into difficulties. It is possible that the Yequana children are able to develop their appreciation of the depth on the basis of an innate fear. The American child was restrained and may have been prevented from acquiring an important experience which he needed for his own protection when exploring. Young children rarely fall down the stairs when they are crawling: they can perceive a change in depth and stop at the top of the stairs. Falling down the stairs is more common when the child begins walking upright, and is a bit clumsy or unsteady. Research at the University of Cambridge has shown that nearly 70% of babies of one to eight months old suffer from astigmatism. This refractive error corrects spontaneously by the time the children are eighteen months old. The explanation for this is not clear but the researchers suggest that normal visual experience causes the eye to regulate its own optics (Atkinson et al 1980). Held et al (1980) have shown that the ability to see in three dimensions first appears at sixteen weeks and develops very rapidly in the following five weeks. Failure to develop proper co-operation between the two eyes at that time is difficult to correct subsequently.

HEARING

Various methods are employed to assess hearing in the newborn. These include the observation of movements, changes in respiration, in electroencephalograph, of skin resistance, cardiac changes and the inhibition of sucking. From a wide range of studies it is clear that normal neonates can appreciate differences in pitch, rhythm, and loudness. The heart rate of babies between one and nine days old has been found to increase in a regular way with an increase in the loudness of a tone (Bartoshuk 1974).

Almost any healthy newborn baby will be aroused by a distinctive sound. The Brazelton Neonatal Behavioural Assessment Score utilizes three kinds of sound to assess not only the infant's ability to hear, but also his ability to learn from what he is hearing. A rattle, a bell and a human voice are used. We have already explained in Chapter 1 how babies differ in their ability to learn about sounds. Some become accustomed to the sound, and show that they can ignore it by not responding (response decrement) quite quickly, and others take much longer. Selecting appropriate signals for attention is an essential part of survival. If too many stimuli attract attention, the individual will be overwhelmed. If too few are used, he may miss an essential one. Habituation is an important process which from birth, and probably before, helps us ignore the repetitive, predictable signals, thereby allowing more time and energy for the new and unusual features of the surrounding world. The normal healthy baby is aroused by the rattle, the bell and the human voice. He may show a general startling, or localised response – such as tight blinking, or respiratory changes. When the baby has settled, the stimulus is presented again, and then after a rest period it is repeated and so on. The fact that, despite individual variations, all babies eventually *shut down* and ignore the stimulus, indicates that they are learning that it is a signal which is irrelevant. Babies can sleep soundly in a place where there is a lot of noise, providing it is a noise to which they have become accustomed. It is the smooth monotony of many lullabies which makes them effective. The unexpected sound produces arousal and wakefulness.

MATURITY OF THE NERVOUS SYSTEM AT BIRTH

Full term normal healthy newborn infants do vary in maturity. Girls, on average, have a more mature nervous system than boys, and it is probably only the more mature infants who are able, in the first two or three weeks, to integrate what they hear with what they see. The orienting reflex – turning to look at a source of sound or movement – so obvious in older children and adults, is not consistently apparent until several months after birth. It has been called the *what's that?* response. A small proportion of babies will turn to look at the source of the human voice. This is very exciting for a mother if her baby turns to look at her when she calls him by name.

A study done at the University of Washington suggest that the neonate can integrate information that comes through different senses. Full-term infants of 26 to 33 days old showed a preference (by looking longer at it) for a shape they had already experienced in the form of a 'pacifier' (an unusual shaped dummy). The researchers conclude that 'neonates are already able to detect tactual-visual correspondences' and 'are capable to using and storing suprisingly abstract information about the objects in their world' (Meltzoff & Borton 1979).

SENSE OF SMELL

Odours are another set of stimuli to which newborn babies will respond. In one study which tested babies on the first, second, third and fourth days of life, for their responsiveness to different concentrations of asafoetida (a gum resin of various oriental plants of the carrot family), it was found that the sensitivity of the babies increased each day, and they were able to respond to smaller concentrations. It is not clear from this whether this improvement in sensitivity is due to maturation or to learning. This increase in sensitivity may seem to contradict our previous comments about response decrement. Response decrement occurs when a single persistent unvarying kind of stimulus is presented. Its monotony and essential lack of significance to the infant, causes the decrease in response. An important feature in the development of heightened sensitivity, is that different stimuli are present, in this case different concentrations, so that the infant has the opportunity of detecting and responding to small changes in his surroundings

A story is told of Ludwig Koch, a naturalist famous for his detailed knowledge of birds and bird song. He was making a recording of an unusual bird song in Regent's Park. When he played his recording back, all that could be heard was the traffic in the Marylebone Road. He had become habituated to the traffic – it was monotonous and of no significance to him – so much so, that he did not recognise its presence. The bird song to which he had become highly sensitised by years of attentive listening to small changes, was all he could hear. The tape recorder had no such selective perception.

A further indication that the infant receives information and learns about his surroundings through his sense of smell, comes from the finding that at two weeks old a baby is more likely to turn his head in the direction of his mother's breast pad than that of any other lactating mother (McFarlane 1975). The mother's smell is one of many stimuli which go to make up the total experience for the baby, of his mother. There are, as has already been mentioned, innumerable interferences between the two while they are in hospital. If smell is important, what effects have the various therapeutic and cosmetic creams and potions which are applied to the nipples and body generally? We do not know. Alterations in the mother's odour may affect the baby's interest in breast feeding as well as his learning about her. Cleaning the areola and the nipple and then applying lanoline is an interference with a natural process which is often avoidable. The sense of smell is more important to many adult animals than it is to adult humans. The area of the brain which is associated with olfaction is in the paleocortex, that part of the cortex which appeared relatively early in the evolution of the brain. The development of the neo-cortex is generally considered to be associated with evolutionary advance in psychomotor and language skills. It is likely that young babies, therefore, depend more than adults on the relatively primitive sense of smell. The possible existence and likely action of human pheromones has been debated in the past few years. A pheromone is an odour which functions as part of a signalling system, and can both arouse and guide behaviour. Pheromonal substances may be released from apocrine glands, axillary secretion or smegma. It has been suggested that pheromones may be important in sexual and social relationships, as well as in infant-parent and child-parent relations (Comfort 1971). It is often found that a particular odour evokes a long past memory with great clarity. The smell of a house in which some childhood holiday was spent, or the scent of a particular person's clothing may set in motion a whole sequence of recollections.

Little research has been done of infants' taste. It is difficult to avoid confusion of taste with smell. Babies do, however, seem to have an established hierarchy of preferences in the order sweet, salt, sour, bitter.

TOUCH AND CONTACT

Babies also experience the world about them through touch, handling, being cuddled, stroked or rocked. Left to themselves mothers will often examine their just born baby by feeling its limbs, stroking it and then cuddling it (Fig. 9.5a & b).

When Harlow separated rhesus monkey babies from their mothers they spent far more time with the soft towelling model in spite of the fact that their food supply was dispensed by the wire one (See Ch. 1). The towelling attracted and satisfied the babies, but when they reached adulthood they had great difficulties in their relationships with other adult rhesus monkeys, and also in caring for their own babies. The towelling mother surrogates did not, of course, handle and carry them in the way a living mother would have done, and they, therefore, had no opportunity to learn important things about their own species.

Mothers and babies who have had the opportunity to experience skin contact for an hour or so after birth have measurable differences in their behaviour, as compared with those who follow the normal hospital routine in which the mother is attended to while the baby is cleaned and dressed elsewhere, put in his cot and sent to the nursery. These studies have already been referred to in Chapter 8 as the extended contact mothers are more likely to persist with breast feeding. They also pay more attention to their babies, and the babies are more advanced by the time they are two years of age.

Many paintings of mothers and babies show the baby being held on the left side of the mother's body. Mother Rhesus monkeys are also more likely to carry their newborn infants on the left. Lee Salk, an American psychologist, has been able to demonstrate in a series of experiments, that in the normal mother and baby relationship, the baby is held on the left side. This applies equally to both left and right handed mothers. He thought this might be because the infant was more peaceful on the left side close to the mother's heart. For nine months he has been developing in close proximity to the aorta. Perhaps, during intrauterine life the infant has learned an association between the rhythmical heart beat, and the protected tension free state. Salk compared two groups of

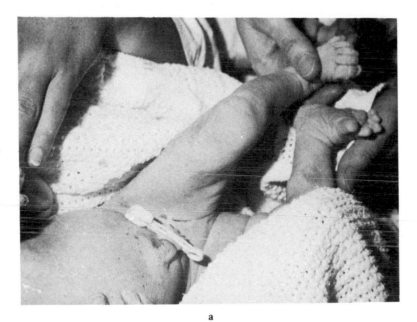

a

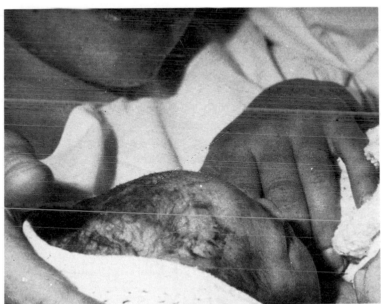

b

Figure 9.5a & 9.5b Mother examining newly born baby by feeling, stroking and cuddling.

newborn infants. One group of 102 babies were placed in a nursery immediately after birth, and were kept there for four days, except for normal feeding by their mothers every four hours. A recording of the sound of an adult heart beat, 72 beats per minute at 85 decibels played continuously day and night. Another group of 112 infants were kept in a quiet nursery. The two groups were compared for weight change and amount of crying. Those infants in the heart beat nursery had a median weight gain of 40 g, and the control group a median loss of 20 g. There were no significant differences in food intake between the two. There was crying for 38 per cent of the time in the heart beat nursery and for 60 per cent of the time in the control group (Fig. 4.6). These results suggest that newborn infants are soothed by the sound of the normal adult heart beat. A recording firm has recently made a record of heart beat sounds which is marketed as a baby soother.

We have come to understand more about the world of the neonate by observing one aspect of his behaviour at a time,

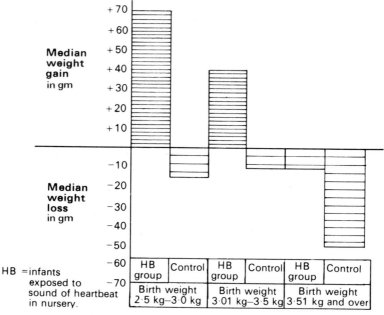

Figure 9.6 Diagram to show effect of recorded adult heart beat on weight gain from 1 to 4 days after birth where amount of feeds were similar (after Salk).

and by presenting him with one isolated stimulus at a time. We can appreciate some of his preferences and predilections. Babies however, normally have to deal with a whole mother – face, colour, sound, smell, heartbeat, nipple, warmth, movement, arms, body – all at once. 'The infant comes well equipped to signal his needs and his gratitude . . . he can . . . make choices about what he wants from his parents and shut out what he doesn't want.' He 'is a powerful force of stabilizing and influencing those around him. . . . we must . . . uncover and expose those infant strengths to parents . . .' (Brazelton 1979). Mother and baby need opportunities for learning about each other as whole human beings, of learning to understand and respond to each other. If they can be assured of these opportunities in the two weeks after birth, they can go home together with more than a satisfactory weight gain for the baby, and an involuted uterus and well healed perineum for the mother. They are likely to have a good foundation for a happy and understanding relationship, which will reduce the risk of acute anxiety which a young mother all too often experiences.

REFERENCES

Atkinson, J., Braddick, O. & French, J. (1980) *Vision Research*, **20** pp 891

Bartoshuk, A. K. (1964) Intensity of Sound. *Psychonomic Science*, **1** pp 151 2.

Brazelton, T. Berry (1979) Earliest Parent-Child Interactions. *Concern*, **22** pp 11–15

Campos, J. J., Langer, A., Krow, A. (1970) *Science*, **170** pp 196–7.

Carpenter, G. C., Tecce, J. J., Stechler, G., Friedman, S (1970) Differential visual behaviour to human and humanoid faces in early infancy. *Merrill Palmer Quarterly*, **16** pp 91 108.

Chase, W. P. (1937) Colour vision in infants. *Journal of Experimental Psychology*, **20** pp 203–322.

Comfort, A. (1971) Likelihood of human pheromones. *Nature*, **230** pp 432–433.

Fantz, R. (1961) *Scientific American*, **204** pp 66–72.

Gibson, E. J. & Walk, R. D. (1960) The visual cliff. *Scientific American*, **202** iv pp 64–71.

Greenman, G. W. (1963) In *Modern perspectives in child development*. Ed. Solnit, A. J. & Provence, S. A. New York: Hallmark.

Haith, M. H. (1972) Visual scanning in infants. In (The Competent Infant, Ed. Stone, L. J., Smith, H. T., & Murphy, L. B. pp 320–323. London: Tavistock Publications.

Held, R., Birch, E., Gwiazda, J. (1980) *Proceedings of the National Academy of Sciences*, **77** pp 5572.

James, W. (1890) *Principles of Psychology*, p 488. New York: Holt.
Korna, A. F. & Grobstein, R. (1966) Visual alertness as related to soothing in neonates. *Child Development*, 37 No. 4 pp 867–876.
Leboyer, F. (1974) *Birth without violence*. London: Wildwood House Ltd.
Leidloff, J. (1975) *The Continuum concept*. London: Duckworth.
McFarlane, J. A. (1975) Olfaction in the development of social preferences in the human neonate. In *Parent-Infant Interaction*. Symposium No. 33, London: CIBA Foundation.
Meltzoff, A. N. & Borton, R. W. (1979) Intermodal matching by human neonates. *Nature*, 282 pp 403–404
Salapatek, P. H. & Kessan, W. (1966) Visual scanning of geometric figures in the human newborn. *Journal of Experimental Child Psychology*, 3 pp 155–167.
Salk, L. (1973) The role of the heartbeat in the relationship between mother and infant. *Scientific American*, 228 pp 24–28.
Wright, P., Crow, R. & Fawcett, G. Personal communication.

10

Development

A midwife's primary concern is the health, comfort and happiness of the mother and baby. Although it is the pregnancy, labour and puerperium which are within the midwife's immediate purview, it is the long term effects of events during that period that are of wider concern.

Babies in some respects are all like – any human infant is distinguishable from any other new born mammal. There are also ways in which a baby is like some other babies. A boy, for example, has some qualities and characteristics in common with all other boys, and these characteristics distinguish him from all girls. There are innumerable criteria for putting people into sub categories. There are also ways in which each baby is a unique individual – his totality of qualities and characteristics that make up his quite distinctive identity.

At conception half the chromosomes from each parent join together to form the first cell, or zygote, of the new individual. The 50 per cent of parental chromosomes which go to the formation of the ovum or the spermatozoon, seems to be largely a matter of chance. From, possibly millions of spermatozoa, only one will fertilise the ovum; which one, is again a matter of chance. Before the zygote has begun to develop the assortment of genetic material is such as to make predictions about the offspring from a knowledge of the parents, something of a gamble. As soon as the ovum has been fertilised, it begins to develop in an environment. The importance of this prenatal environment is discussed in the chapter about antenatal events.

NATURE OR NURTURE?

Almost every individual varies in his genetic endowment and his experiences. If two factors vary at the same time, it is impossible to find out which one is responsible for an observed difference. Is a child good at mathematics because he has an inborn aptitutde (heredity) or because he has had special training e.g. a particularly good teacher (environment), or because his inherited predisposition and experience have interacted in an advantageous way? In the case of one individual, it is often impossible to say how far a particular characteristic is derived from environmental factors and how far from heredity. The nature-nurture issue has been the subject of endless debate. 'What's born in the blood comes out in the bone' is a saying supporting the *nature* side of the argument while ' as the twig is bent so the tree grows' supports the *nurture* side. This is an issue of great importance to everyone who has anything to do with child care. If development depends primarily on *nature* then variations in *nurture* will have relatively little impact. Much of the endeavour in the biological and behavioural sciences, have been directed to finding out what changes in *nurture*, do, or can affect development. Improvements in obstetrics, in baby feeding, in special provisions for small, preterm or sick babies have all helped to reduce the infant mortality rate, and to reduce morbidity.

What do we know of the factors which can affect long term happiness, achievement, learning ability, concentration, ability to think and reflect, self assurance, anxiety, which are also of such importance in good physical and mental health? These psychological features, and many more, are derived from either *nature*, or *nurture*, or are a product of some interaction between the two.

ENVIRONMENTAL INFLUENCES ON DEVELOPMENT

Psychologists have tried to tease out some answers to these questions by a number of different methods. Experiments with animals can sometimes provide important clues and ideas, but it is wrong to extrapolate from animal studies to human beings as if they are much alike. The response of human beings to any experience is complicated by their use of language and their complex social structure.

The question of the effect of fetal environment on development is dealt with in detail in the chapter on antenatal events. The way in which the fetus develops may have long term consequences for the development of the child. The uterine environment may give rise to subtle changes which though causing no macroscopic abnormality, may somehow affect the developing neural tissues of the fetus which govern behaviour in later life. De Licardie and Cravioto (1974) have shown how poor diet affects long term development and intellectual achievement. The National Child Development Study has found that children of mothers who smoked during the pregnancy have a depressed reading age at seven years (Davie et al 1972). Hypoxia may affect brain tissue extensively, producing long term problems such as subnormality, clumsiness, speech defects, poor motor coordination and behaviour problems. Chronic hypoxia may be caused by placental insufficiency of unknown aetiology, or that associated with hypertension, renal disease, and other adverse factors. The long term effects for the child, the family and the community, of these very early events are of great consequence. One of the trials of life is that the poor conditions during pregnancy which contribute towards difficulties in the offspring, are more common in lower working class families, who are least able to contend with the additional strain imposed by a less-than-whole child.

Identical (uniovular) twins have been studied quite extensively. They provide a natural occurring situation in which inherited factors are constant, as they have developed from a single zygote. Identical twins, however, normally grow up in the same family, and experience very similar environments. Occasionally identical twins are separated. Such separated uniovular twins have been the basis of a few important studies of development, as they provide conditions in which one of the variables in the important nature-nurture equation is the same. Observed differences between the twins may reasonably be attributed to differences in their background, upbringing, experiences – in short, to their *nurture*.

A further method is to assess the effects of either enhancing or depriving a group of chlidren of an experience, and comparing them with another group who have not been so treated. The intentional deprivation of a group of children for scientific purposes would, needless to say, be unethical, but there are plenty of spontaneously occurring deprivations the effects of which can be, and have been, assessed. Intentional enhancement is often severely frowned upon as well, as it is considered improper to provide a supposed advantage to one but not to all.

Several of the sources of information already referred to in this book are based on ethological studies. Ethology first emerged in the 1950s, as the study of animal behaviour, and was concerned with the detailed observation of behaviour which occurred naturally in the normal habitat. The first ethologists were critical of the *experimental laboratory* approach to behaviour, which required the animal (or human) to perform a sequence of behaviour which was often quite foreign to him under artifical conditions. Ethological studies of child behaviour are those in which careful observations are made of the child, or mother and child in the course of their normal daily life, for example – what does a mother do when her baby cries? The answer to that question probably has an important bearing on how the infant develops socially and emotionally. By noting carefully, sometimes with the aid of a videotaped recording, how a number of mothers and babies behave with each other, it has been possible to come to some general conclusions about particular aspects of child development. In this chapter we shall refer to information culled from the study of subhuman mammals, twins, groups of children who have been enhanced or deprived of particular experiences, and from ethological studies.

DEPRIVATIONS

A number of apocryphal stories about feral children reared by animals exist. There are few properly documented accounts of the development of children grossly deprived of any sort of human contact. Those which do exist make it plain that many of the qualities and traits we regard as characteristically human are learned; the upright posture, speech, the communicative gesture and facial expressions need either example or precept to emerge. In the absence of facilitative experience the inborn capacity for a whole range of behaviour remains dormant.

Many years ago Jean-Marc-Gaspard Itard published an account of his attempts to humanise a boy who had lived wild in the woods around Paris. *The Wild Boy of Aveyron* is one of the earliest studies of the effect of environment on growth and behaviour.

Fortunately such bizarre experiences are extremely rare. Children brought up in institutions usually have a background distinctively different from that of children in families, and have been the subject of concern for almost a century. Published figures in Europe and America showed that in the first two decades of this century the mortality rate of infants reared in institutions was extremely high – between 30 per cent and 100 per cent. By the 1940s this high mortality rate had been reduced, and was in line with that of the general population. With the survival of institutionalised children a new problem emerged. '. . . Institutionalised children, practically without exception developed subsequent psychiatric disturbances and became a social, delinquent, feeble minded, psychotic and problem children.' In this country the recommendations of the Curtis Report on the care of children deprived of a normal home life (Report on the Care of Children Committee 1947) and Bowlby's report for the World Health Organisation drew attention to some of the important factors which seemed to the authors to contribute to intellectual, emotional and social difficulties of infants and children in orphanages and foundling homes. Institutional life is usually characterised by impersonal relationships, regimentation, an emphasis on order, cleanliness and discipline. Children reared in families grow up, by and large, without the problems which beset a considerable proportion of those reared in institutions. This broad comparison of two large groups of children led to specific conclusions and recommendations. The Curtis Report recommended fostering for young children, where possible. Where it was not possible, a more homely atmosphere, with smaller groups of children, and an identifiable house parent was advocated. Bowlby identified the source of the problem for children in institutions as that of being deprived of their mother. He claimed that a warm, continuous, and intimate relationship with his mother, or a mother surrogate, was essential for the child's good mental health. Bowlby has been the single most important influence on thinking about the child's mental development in this country. Many of the cruder effects on children of going to hospital and into children's homes, can now be ameliorated, if opportunities are provided for visiting, and for the maintenance or cultivation of a close personal affectionate relationship. It is a measure of the success of Bowlby's proselytising that everyone now seems to recognise, that as well as food and warmth, an infant needs loving care and attention. For comparison look at some of the child care manuals published before the 1940s. Their emphasis was mainly on feeding, cleanliness, and discipline and order. Affectionate attention by parents was seldom mentioned and sometimes regarded a sign of moral turpitude.

BONDING OR ATTACHMENT

The importance of a loving relationship between mother and child leads, according to Bowlby, to *bonding* between the two. In later writing, Bowlby (1969) has used the term *attachment* in place of *bonding*. The attachment to an adult of the species, is an important feature in the development of the young, of a large number of birds and animals, as has been discovered by the ethologists. A lot of species-appropriate behaviour can be learned from the adult to whom the infant becomes attached. In quite normal families infants may develop multiple attachments. or they may be devoted to an adult other than their mother. Some youngster become specially devoted to an older sibling, their father, or a grandmother for example. What does seem to be of great importance is that the person or persons with whom a particular affection is developed, should maintain the relationship. One of the damaging experiences in institutional homes derived, and still does, from the fact that staff so frequently change and special attachments have little opportunity to flourish.

The first two years of life is a period during which affectionate attachment for one, or a few people, develops with ease if the infant is lovingly cared for and attended. Some psychologists disapprove of the term *attachment* as it suggests an almost mechanical relationships – like being tied together with a rope. Any mechanical analogy of this sort may mask the important fact that the relationship is essentially a social one, which depends on subtle signals and learning for its development. How readily a satisfactory and rewarding relationship can develop later on, if it fails to do so in the early years, is still a matter of debate. What does seem reasonably clear is that the first experiences of other people who are important in the infant's world, form something of a prototype for subsequent encounters. If the initial experiences are uncomfortable and unrewarding those which follow are not embarked upon with trust and social ease.

Children learn from their parents and caretakers, but so do parents learn from their children. A mother with a new baby often looks and feels ill at ease because she has no experience in interpreting what the needs of the child are, and does not know how to handle him. She learns a great deal by noticing what he likes and dislikes. The process whereby the parents and siblings become attached to the new member of the family, are perhaps as important as the process by which he becomes attached to them.

Affection, security, warmth, continuity, intimacy, describe positive emotional qualities of a relationship. The child who experiences them is likely to develop similar qualities. As a child grows older he will want to explore, to try out his own abilities, and to find things out for himself. Finding out about his surroundings – what they are made of, how they work, and so on, form an important part of the child's intellectual development. Children who are emotionally insecure are easily frightened. Easily frightened children don't explore. Children who don't explore don't learn. So having a good relationship which generates a feeling of security is important, not only for emotional well-being, but has an important bearing on the way a child builds up a store of knowledge about the world.

INNATE FACTORS

There are a number of features which affect the emotional stability, in addition to the sort of relationship the infant enjoys in early life. There is good evidence that emotionality is in part innate (Shields 1962). On long term study which followed children from birth to ten shows how persistent emotional characteristics assessed at birth are (Thomas et al 1970). The tendency to be excitable or placid, shows at or soon after birth. Babies, like adults, vary in the speed at which they habituate. This variation is made use of in the Brazelton Assessment Scale of Neonatal Abilties (see Ch. 9).

A young baby explores with his eyes, later with his hands, and as soon as he can crawl or walk, he becomes vigorously active in his search for novelty. An attempt has been made to account for changes in interest and attention, by the discrepancy hypothesis which runs thus:

> When faced with a new stimulus we match it against information we already have stored in our memory. If the new stimulus exactly fits a stored image or memory, little interest is aroused – it is entirely predictable and boring. If it is very different from the stored memory, it is too novel, alarming, and arouses fear, and thus inhibits curiosity. It is the stimulus with some recognisable, and also some novel features, which maximises curiosity and exploration.

These three separate factors, innate emotionality, early experience, and the degree of novelty in a situation will affect the interest, and attention, a child can devote to his surroundings, and hence the amount he can learn. The child who fidgets, is unable to concentrate and is easily distractable, usually has a difficult time at school, and compares unfavourably with the youngster who is able to approach a new problem with interested concentration. An important dimension which emerges in children of school age is that of reflectivity and impulsiveness (Kagan & Freeman 1963).

The reflective child when faced with a problem thinks before acting or speaking, whereas the impulsive one tries an immediate solution to the problem, fails, is upset by his failure, and makes further impulsive attempts becoming more and more frustrated.

It is by no means far fetched to suggest that the midwife may have an important part to play in the long term emotional and intellectual development of the normal babies for whom she cares. (The small, ill or handicapped infants are discussed in Chapter 6.) Variations in innate emotionality cannot be altered. Some babies will be by nature more restless, will cry more and be more difficult to settle than others. These babies will need more skilled handling and patience, and their mothers, especially the inexperienced, may not be very good initially, at providing this. A midwife may be able to give an example to an inexperienced mother and also to help her to keep calm and patient. Placid babies usually make for placid mothers and the converse is also true. Any midwife who can help to introduce stability and calm into the relationship, may make a valuable contribution to the baby's long-term development.

As has been mentioned elsewhere, Richards (1975) has shown that the pattern of crying is a relatively persistent characteristic of a baby, and it is important, therefore, that the mother is not made to feel she is mishandling him. It may be necessary to acknowledge the fact that the baby is *not* going to turn into a placid peaceful child, and to help the mother adjust *her* life to accord with the infant's needs. The mother of a fidgeting or fretful baby, is likely to be grateful for months ahead for any help, example, or encouragement which leads to her more successful adjustment to the infant.

STIMULATION

Ideally everyone has an optimal degree of arousal at which learning is maximised. Insufficient arousal induces apathy and a lack of awareness; excessive arousal means too much anxiety and emotion, which can be disruptive. Learning requires not only a suitable state in the learner, but something *out there* to be learned. A dull environment is likely to make a dull child. Young animals who have been reared with things to play with, turn out to be more intelligent than similar litter mates who have only been able to *look* at the play objects, and they in turn are brighter than animals who have had no opportunity to *feel* or *see* a variety of objects (Forgus 1966).

It is now a truism that children who have the benefit of a more stimulating environment, generally develop into brighter people. A stimulating environment means one which provides a wide range of experiences with things to look at, hear, touch, and with opportunities for exploration, manipulation, and play with things and people. The abilities of the newborn are considerably more advanced than many people have supposed. In order to develop an ability it needs opportunity for exercise. It follows, therefore, that if an infant can distinguish shapes, colour and pattern, an opportunity for development is being missed if he cannot visually explore such things. Fantz (1966) has found that he can distinguish babies who have been brought up in an institution from those who are reared at home, by their visual responses at two months old. Babies cared for by their own mothers are probably exposed to a richer visual environment as they are picked up more often and have the chance to look round. The long term consequences of this, of course, are not known, but the first two months of life is only lived through once. It is from this kind of detailed study, that the precise meaning of institutional deprivation begins to be clarified.

LANGUAGE

Another area of experience, which is of powerful importance in intellectual development, is in language learning. We need words to describe and communicate our experiences, but they also help us to make perceptual discriminations. We probably all have some practical experience of this fact if we recall the process of some new learning. In midwifery for example, we used to learn about the premature baby. The concept of prematurity we now know confuses two different problems namely, pre-term birth and slow intra-uterine growth. Both result in a low birth weight baby. The more discriminating perception of pre-term-ness and small-for-dates-ness required new words as labels. These words, in turn, help a student to perceive differences between the two kinds of baby. The distinction between the two has led to improvements in treatment and prognosis. The perception, and the word-label which denotes it are closely associated together.

Much education depends on a refinement of perception. In advanced society, education at all levels proceeds mainly by teaching – through the spoken or written word. This is in contrast to primitive societies where education procedes by showing, and the learner is immediately involved in the task situation of, say hunting or cooking. This means that achievement and satisfactions, in an advanced society, not only within the educational system, but in life generally, are very likely to be associated with good linguistic and verbal abilities. Children do not normally speak their first words until they are about a year old. As anyone who has learned a foreign language can readily appreciate, however, there is a distinction between passive and active language. Passive language refers to the considerable understanding which usually precedes the ability to speak. Institutional children, it has been found, have fewer words in their repertoire than have home reared children. Well before any question of words or language arises, there are measurable differences in, not only the number of sounds which the two groups of children make, but the number of times they make them (Irwin 1949).

DIFFERENT TYPES OF THINKING

From within a few days or weeks of birth, vocalisation is encouraged by the mother who talks to or answers her child when he makes a sound, which includes crying. The infant who burbles and cries and receives no *sound* in reply, is less likely to continue sound making, and also less able to learn different kinds of sound. Innumerable follow-up studies of infants both normal and disadvantaged at birth, testify to the fact that the socio-economic position of the families in which they are reared, is of overwhelming importance to their long term development. In what way does the home of the higher social class child differ from that of the lower class child? To generalise from a number of studies it is clear that middle class mothers engage in much more verbal interaction, (Levine et al 1967, Tulkin & Kagan 1972) and working class parents provide more physical stimulation for their infants (Moss et al 1969). No substantial difference between the classes has been established so far as affective (emotional) behaviour is concerned (Bayley & Shaefer 1960, Kagan & Freeman 1963). Middle class parents seem to provide a greater variety of stimulation, and markedly more verbal variety. It is important to recognise that these variations are part of traditional culture. They show that different groups of people within society have characteristic way of behaving and communicating with each other. Cultural patterns and traditions have developed to meet some important need, or in response to a particular environment. Intellectual development and school achievement are both heavily dependent on symbolic activity, and *telling type* instructions. The use of word and number enables the user to refer to, and think about, objects and ideas which are not immediately present. A symbol stands for something other than itself, and the use of symbols greatly enriches our potential for thinking and communicating. It enables us to talk about things that are far distant in space and time, enabling us to bring the past and future into present discourse. Bruner distinguishes between three kinds of thinking. Enactive thinking is that which goes on in muscles, joints and brain when for example, we ride a bicycle, swim or walk upstairs. Most of us would not call this thinking at all. These are, however, activities which have been learned, and information about how to do them is stored somewhere in the nervous system. Iconic thinking is that which goes on when we imagine things – our living room at home, the play we saw last night, the first delivery we witnessed. These are *pictures in the head* which can be experienced quite independently of words. To be able to communicate the experience with any accuracy we need the third kind of thinking, namely, symbolic thinking which depends upon the translation of an image or idea into a symbol. In order to communicate anything about last night's play, or the first delivery we witnessed, we need to be able to translate details of the image into symbols such as stage, actor, etc. In adulthood we engage at various times in enactive, iconic and symbolic thinking, but the ability to do so is a consequence of development. It is often found that practical people who can 'see how to do things' are not very good at instructing anyone else. The instruction may require translating from iconic to symbolic thinking.

Nurses often learn the requirements for a particular procedure from a trolley diagram. The equipment for a lumbar puncture or intravenous infusion is often presented in visual terms and is remembered iconically. Images are relatively inflexible and they can be retained without any real understanding of the purpose of the parts. An alternative method of learning about the requirements for a lumbar puncture and so on, is to use symbolic thinking. This requires some discussion of the technical process involved and an understanding of the necessary steps to perform it. Every trolley need not look exactly alike – what is required is a collection of containers, fluids, swabs, local anaesthetic and the means of administering it all arranged in such a way as to have regard to asepsis, comfort of the patient and so on. Symbolic thinking enables the nurse to be much more adaptable.

The newborn child's experience of his surroundings is probably mainly enactive – bodily sensations and experiences. Babies of two weeks old have shown by their behaviour that they can remember something about their mother's face (Carpenter 1974), and also that they can remember how far away an object was from them (Bower 1974). This seems to indicate that even very young children have the beginnings of iconic thinking.

There remain many unanswered questions about long term development of skills, abilities, inventiveness and ingenuity, mental health, contentment, assurance and sociability. It is, however, now reasonably clear that development depends upon information and experiences that get in from the outside, as well as the unfolding of potential from the inside. There is good evidence that development of cognitive ability (that is to think, reason, understand, etc.) is as much from the *outside in*, as from the *inside out*. The midwife is present at the beginning, and by the experiences she is able to provide, and the discussion she is able to have with the mother, may be an important influence in what passes from the *outside in*.

SPECIAL CARE BABY UNITS

Babies who are nursed in intensvie special care units may have particular problems arising out of their isolation (Fig. 10.1). Babies in incubators experience a different quality of care and human contact, from that of a well full term baby. They have less close physical contact, do not experience a diurnal rhythm of light and darkness, hear unusual and monotonous sounds which rarely include the human voice, have a greater variety of caretakers and a wider range of tactile and painful experiences.

Little is known at present of the abilities of the pre-term infant, that is, what he can see, hear, remember and what he selects for attention and so on. It is likely that these abilities need time to develop, but we do not know. It has been shown that the contact between mothers and their babies in incubators is remarkably slight, even when visiting is encouraged (Prince et al 1978). The midwife who is caring for such babies may be able to provide more normal experiences for them and, above all, encouraging their parents to do likewise. Little will be lost if their neurological apparatus is insufficiently mature to hear or see stimuli which are provided.

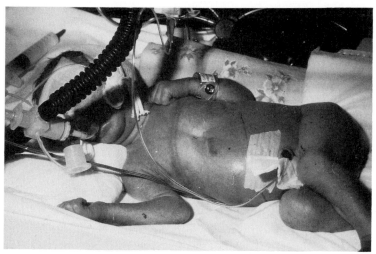

Figure 10.1 Baby in incubator, isolated from usual human contact.

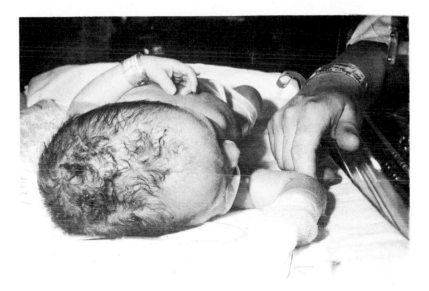

Figure 10.2 A sick baby being given extra tactile, visual and kinaesthetic stimulation.

Their development may be unnecessarily hampered by an absence of stimulation. An experiment in which pre-term babies were given extra tactile, visual, and kinaesthetic stimulation compared very favourably in weight gain and behavioural development with controls who were not so treated (Scarr-Salapatek & Williams 1973) (Fig. 10.2). Other problems associated with small pre-term and ill babies are discussed in Chapter 11. The midwife can play a very important role here in ensuring that contact by parents, and the level and type of stimulation is maintained near to the normal pattern as is compatible with the high standards of physical care so vital to his healthy survival.

REFERENCES

Bayley, N. & Shaefer, E. (1960) *Journal of Genetic Psychology*, **96** pp 61–77.
Bower, T. (1974) Competent Newborns. *New Scientist*, **61** pp 672.
Bowlby, J. (1951) *Maternal Care and Mental Health*, Monograph 3 Geneva: WHO.
Bowlby, J. (1969) Attachment. *Attachment & Loss*, Vil. I. London: Hogarth Press.

Carpenter, G. (1974) Mother's Face and the Newborn. *New Scientist,* **61** pp 742.

Davie, R., Butler, N., Goldstein, J. H. (1972) *From Birth to Eleven.* Harlow: Longmans for the National Children's Bureau.

de Licardie, E. R. & Cravioto, J. (1974) Behavioural responsiveness of survivors of clinical severe malnutrition to cognitive demands, in *Early Malnutrition and Mental Development.* Ed. by Cravioto, J., Hambraeus, L., Vahl Guist, B. Swedish Nutrition Foundation.

Fantz, R. L. F. (1966) The Crucial Early Influence: Mother love or environmental stimulation? *American Journal of Orthopsychiatry,* **36** No. 2. pp 330–336.

Forgus, R. H. (1966) *Perception: The Basic Process in Cognitive Development.* New York: McGraw Hill.

Irwin, O. C. (1949) Infant Speech *Scientific American,* **181** pp 22–24.

Jean-Marc-Gaspard Itard (1962) *The Wild Boy of Aveyron,* translated by George & Muriel Humphrey. New York: Appleton Century Crofts.

Kagan, J. & Freeman, M. (1963) *Child Development,* **34** pp 899–911.

Levine, J., Fishman, O. & Kagan, J. (1967) *Society for Research in Child Development.*

Moss, H. A., Robson, K. S. & Pederson, F. (1969) *Developmental Psychology,* **239**–246.

Prince, J., Firlej, M., Harvey, D. (1978) Contact between babies in incubators and their caretakers. In *Early Separation and Special Care Nurseries,* Ed. Brimblecombe, F. S. W., Richards, M. P. M., Robertson, N. R. C. London: Heinemann Medical Books.

Report on the Care of Children Committee: *The Curtis Report* (1947) London: HMSO.

Richards, M. P. M. (1975) Unpublished lecture delivered at St Charles' Hospital, Ladbroke Grove.

Scarr-Salapatek, S. & Williams, M. L. (1973) The Effects of Early Stimulation on Low-Birth Weight Infants. *Child Development,* **44** (1) pp 94–101.

Shields, R. (1962) *Monozygotic Twins.* Oxford: Oxford University Press.

Spitz, R. A. (1945) Hospitalisation. An enquiry into the genesis of psychiatric conditions in early childhood. *Psychoanalytic study of the child,* **1** pp 57–74. New York: International Universities Press.

Thomas, A., Chess, S. & Birch, H. (1970) 'The Origin of Personality'. *Scientific American,* **223** (2) pp 102–109.

Tulkin, S. & Kagan, J. (1972) *Child Development,* **43** 30–41.

Handicaps

A handicap for a runner in a race is an advantage conferred, or an adverse condition imposed, so that the chances of the competitors are made more nearly equal. An adverse condition, extra weight to be carried, or a delay in starting, is imposed on an individual who has shown evidence of being particularly good. Although the term can be used to mean an advantage, it is more generally applied to the imposition of a disadvantage. Conditions referred to as *handicapping* in infants and children, are always those which seem to weaken the child's chance of survival, or make a satisfactory adaptation to life more difficult. An extremely attractive appearance, or exceptionally high intelligence are not generally regarded as handicaps, although they may militate against satisfactory adaptation in society. Many characteristics of individuals are distributed normally throughout the population, that is to say, most people are to be found in the middle ranges and comparatively few at the low or high end. Take height for example – the average height of 18 year old boys is, at present, 174 cm; very few are less than 160 cm and very few more than 190 cm. Young men at the extremes are faced with a number of difficulties of which their peers of more average height know nothing. They will find it more difficult to buy clothes that they like to fit them, and they will have to pay more for them. The clothing manufacturers mass produce for the average. Social relations may not be so easy either. The short boy may be treated as if he were younger and less capable than he feels – the opposite is true for the very tall. In social relations height is important. Someone we have to look up to in a physical sense is spontaneously attributed with authority and dominance. The short man cannot assume an authoritative role but has to assert himself to achieve it.

DEVIATION FROM THE NORM

The values, standards, ideals and customs of a culture can usually be found to be derived from the norms of that culture. Individuals too far away in either direction from the norm are likely to experience some kind of social pressure. The exceptionally quick learner is often as much of a problem for the teacher in the classroom, as the exceptionally slow one. There are many examples in history of innovatory ideas appearing *before their time* – that is, being too far away from the social and intellectual norms of the time. Advantages and disadvantages have, therefore, to be seen in relation to the norms and values which are generally held in society. It must be remembered also, that these do change – sometimes fairly quickly. A glance through a fashion magazine of 20 or 30 years ago readily shows how ephemeral notions of beauty are.

The survival rate of handicapped infants has increased, together with the general improvement in infant survival rate. Furthermore, medical advances ensure that many survive into adulthood, and may indeed have an average expectation of life. Whether social attitudes and values have changed commensurately to accommodate a wider range of characteristics and abilities is a matter of conjecture. There are a number of hopeful signs. There is a genuine interest in, and attempt to make provision for, care in the community rather than in an institution. Community care for a child with Down's syndrome for example, is likely to mean care by the family with support from local health and social services, both statutory and voluntary. Inadequacy of this support may contribute to a family succumbing, and the child becoming institutionalised. How far local support is forthcoming will depend on prevailing social attitudes as well as central policies.

HANDICAP IN A SOCIAL CONTEXT

Discussions and decisions within the hospital about a handicapped baby do need to take into account social policies and conditions outside the hospital. One family may have the material, psychological and spiritual resources to rear unaided a handicapped child, and help him achieve his full potential, whereas another would flounder under such a burden. Some knowledge of local provision is, therefore, essential. Different ethnic and social groups not only have some handicapping conditions which are either peculiar, or more common to them (e.g. Tay-Sachs amongst Jews, spina bifida amongst the Irish) but also probably have specialised attitudes which so far as we can discover have not been the subject of any detailed study. For example in a social group which depends on a good physique for its survival – perhaps a primitive agricultural community – physical handicaps such as talipes or congenital dislocation of the hip, may cause more consternation than mental handicap. A short film called Michael (BFI 1960) shows how happily a boy with Down's syndrome fits into rural farm life in Suffolk. On the other hand, a child with a poor physique but good intellect is likely to experience favourable attitudes in an intellectual and bookish family. It has been shown that some Africans use their bodies in movement and gesture to communicate, more than Europeans do. Clumsiness and psychomotor disabilities are likely to be more apparent, and of greater social significance in such a society than in one where communication depends more on language.

The medical view of a handicap is usually coloured by its long term prognosis, the amount of surgical correction entailed and the course of treatment and management envisaged. A parent's response to an ill or disabled baby may be determined by quite different factors, and it may be helpful here to classify handicaps by criteria other than those normally used in paediatric literature.

Sometimes a mother is aware that there is a risk of her baby being born small or before full term. Her own experience, if she has had previous children, may make her suspicious but it is more likely that she will be aware of the concern that is conveyed, directly or otherwise, by obstetrician or midwife. By no means all mothers realise the implications for the baby of low birth weight. Even if she is not surprised by an early delivery she may nevertheless be unprepared for the possibility of her baby being ill. Mothers of multiple births similarly are sometimes not prepared for small babies. Even so, no one can predict with any accuracy the condition of the baby, or babies, and the drama of the birth is likely to be heightened by the hopes and anxieties that surround it.

TYPES OF HANDICAP

About one baby in 40 is born with some kind of handicap. This may be a visible defect, or a disease which is not immediately apparent, for example, cystic fibrosis. The handicap may shorten his expectation of life and may affect his prospects for physical and mental development.

Parents do not always assess their baby by the same criteria as health professionals. A malformation which a paediatrician may regard as easily remediable, may seem quite appalling to the mother and father. On the other hand, the high risk of imminent death associated with some few abnormalities, may not be recognised by the parents unless they are given some special help to come to a realistic appreciation of the fact. One of the authors has had the unhappy experience of trying to convey to a father the seriousness of his baby's respiratory distress. Despite considerable endeavour in emphasising the gravity of the situation, and a refusal to recognise his alternative proposal that 'The baby will be alright', he seemed quite unable to take in such bad news. He was shocked and angry when the baby died. Sometimes the inability to acknowledge the disaster extends further, and the dead baby is treated as if it were still alive. Anthropologists have found in some cultures where babies are carried on the body, that a dead child is carried by the mother until it stinks.

DEVELOPMENT OF HANDICAPPED CHILDREN

There is a considerable amount of evidence that handicapped and unusual children, like their normal brothers and sisters, develop emotionally, socially and intellectually better in a family than in an institution. This fact should not lead us to overlook or minimise the problems which some handicapped children can create for their families, perhaps especially the mother. Events in the immediate postnatal period are of crucial importance, but they must be seen as part of a continuing process in which practical advice and help, as well as support and understanding are available from other professions and services to the family of the handicapped child. It is undoubtedly highly desirable for the child that he should have the opportunity of growing up in an affectionate and caring family setting. Should his parents be unable to accept him as an individual who needs their concern and consideration, or even worse, if he is entirely rejected, this can but add a further handicap with which he must contend.

Careful consideration, therefore, needs to go into the question of communicating with the parents in the postnatal period. Disfigurements of the face cannot be hidden and the mother is immediately aware of them. Physical appearance is an important element in interpersonal relations, and in the last two decades there have been several studies demonstrating the psychological importance of physical appearance (Clifford & Bull 1976). Many mothers, especially first mothers, have built up a picture of the lovely baby they are going to have from pictures, advertisements and a selection of the prettiest or most handsome of older children they know. A baby with a large strawberry naevus, port-wine stain, cleft palate and cleft lip, or some other facial disfigurement, may shock the mother deeply (Figs. 11.1 & 11.2). It may be doubly important for such a mother to hold her baby and to feel him. She may not want to look at him, but the early post-partum contact which has been shown to be so important for the development of good relations between mother and baby (Kennell & Klaus 1972) can be through tactile experience and bodily contact.

Prospects for repair and correction involving medical and surgical decisions and procedures, will be discussed with the

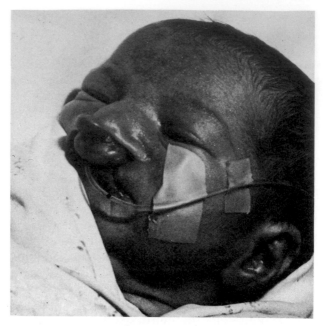

Figure 11.1. Baby with a cleft lip.

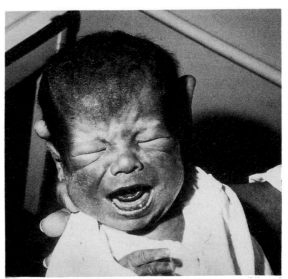

Figure 11.2. Baby with a damaged face.

parents as far as is practicable. The possibilities and likely outcome and plans for treatment, will be communicated by the paediatrician or surgeon. Further discussions by the midwife of what has been said by them may be very helpful to the mother. She may have neither taken in, nor fully understood what has been said. There may be questions which she is apprehensive of putting to the medical staff and undoubtedly she will forget much of what is explained, and communication about the baby, his treatment and future must be a continuing process between staff and both parents. The mother is likely to have many questions to ask and many more for which she cannot find the words. They may remain as amorphous worries which cannot be readily crystalised into language.

HELPING THE MOTHER OF A HANDICAPPED BABY

A midwife who has built up a relationship with the mother may, if she can spend time with her, learn much about her feelings. This will involve not only listening to what is said, but being aware of the significance of many non-verbal communications. Non-verbal signals can be very subtle. There are the questions and comments which never receive a reply, or which occasion a change of topic. Slight changes of expression, about the mouth and eyes, especially the making or evading of eye contact, convey something of the type and intensity of feeling. A change of posture, a seemingly irrel-event gesture can signal intent, confusion, despair or satis-faction. It often seems to be forgotten in hospital, that communication with someone in bed, is facilitated by sitting by the bed and being within a range of about two feet. The midwife who stands over a patient is in an authoritative position and will be treated as such. Authorities on the whole tell, they do not listen. Patients often say they have not talked to sister because she always seems so busy. This apparent lack of time for talking is often eloquently conveyed by the speed at which people walk. Compare, for example, walking speeds of patients, nursing and medical staff.

A mother's feelings in the puerperium may vitally affect the way in which she handles and manages her baby. These may be of grief for the image of the beautiful normal baby who has not been born to her. There may be anger, depression, guilt, self criticism, aggressive feelings towards the hospital, the midwife or the baby himself. Anger is sometimes strongly expressed by the father. Some of the visually distressing handicaps can be effectively corrected. Extra fingers, bat ears, cleft lip, however, may affect the amount of contact the mother is willing to make with her child in the post-partum period. The infant has a number of ways by which he attracts the mother and keeps in touch with her. Sucking, clinging and following with the eyes, are apparent at birth of shortly afterwards. By these means he can maintain contact with his mother. By crying and smiling he can attract her attention. The way the mother responds to the activities is important for the development of attachment behaviour. The midwife can do much to encourage this. The feeding difficulties of the baby with a cleft lip and cleft palate may distort sucking behaviour, as limb defects may distort clinging. Sometimes a baby with a cleft lip can breast feed satisfactorily, and it is well worth encouraging the mother to try this. The mother may inadvertently add further difficulties to the baby's development of a repertoire of social and attachment behaviour by being unwilling to look at him. Despite these difficulties, however, babies with visible facial defects are very rarely rejected. Most parents will know someone who has had a successful repair so there is good reason to be hopeful.

A study of the psychological effects of facial deformity in children (Lansdown & Polok 1975) shows that children of school age are remarkably consistent in their judgements of facial malformations. 75 children aged 9–11 in London and Amsterdam consistently judged as least favourable – protruding teeth, next cleft lip, squint, misshapen nose, and bat ears, in that order. In the same study 24 children who had been operated on for correction of cleft lip in 1965 were followed up. Their behaviour and attainment were compared with that of normal children. They were all 7 or 8 years old. On neither of these measures were there any significant differences. One inference to be drawn is that children disadvantaged in their appearance may have compensated by the development of other valued qualities and characteristics. This phenomenon of compensation in not unusual but it does require cultivation, and the parents are the most likely people to be able to encourage it. It is important, therefore, when discussing the baby with the parents to be quite clear that he has, like any other human being, a great variety of needs, for which he is dependent on his parents, and a wealth of potentialities and capacities which require suitable opportunities for their development.

Some authorities are of the opinion that the father is often better able to take a long term view and a more objective approach to the problem of an abnormal baby, while the mother is more likely to be disproportionately concerned with immediacies. Experienced workers with whom we have discussed this have rarely found this to be so. Some fathers, particularly from cultures where the male retains his dominant position in society, feel an abnormal baby to be an unfavourable comment on their manhood. There will, however, in most cases be two parents with whom the midwife is in regular communication. One may help the other, or they may confuse one another. They may be better able to talk things over about their baby in the presence of a third person. Broaching a sensitive topic can be difficult for two people on their own. If embarrassment, or anger is aroused, the only path open to them may be to terminate the interaction. A third person can be used as a sounding board or as someone to hold the balance. A communication which might be difficult for one parent to make directly to the other can be facilitated by being apparently said to the third person. We all make use of this social facilitation and are usually unaware of doing so.

A task of primary importance is that of enabling the parents to develop a close affectionate relationship with their baby. An acknowledgement of the baby as someone with many positive qualities, and of the parents as being responsible and capable, with help, of nurturing these qualities, may go far to achieve that task.

THE SERIOUSLY ILL BABY

Further difficulties are raised by the baby who has some visible defect which is unlikely to be remediable. Malforma-

tions of the central nervous system, spina bifida, hydrocephalus, anencephalus come into this group. In addition to the
immediate blow to the hope of having a whole and attractive
baby, the parents have an indeterminate period of uncertainty
as to the length and quality of the child's life. Parents facing
the prospect of caring for a child of limited physical and
mental capacity, not only need great personal resources, but
all the help they can get from agencies in the community to
which they can be introduced before they go home. The
isolated and unsupported family is the one which is most
likely to succumb to the strain of having a handicapped child.
A study by Sheila Hewett (1970) of families of handicapped
children in the East Midlands, shows the conflict which is
sometimes experienced when professional workers can do
nothing of a practical nature. One mother referring to the
health visitor, said, 'I was absolutely longing to talk to somebody and every time she came up the road I thought, "Surely
she's coming to see me *this* time" – I think she would he
helpful if she could . . . but there's nothing they can say'. This
is one of many examples given where both mother and
professional worker see the *real job* as taking some specific
action. Where there is no solution to the problem, and health
professionals are sometimes embarrassed at having to
acknowledge their inadequacy, contacts are then awkward
and tend to be avoided. The patient with a terminal illness in
a ward is generally the one most avoided. Yet it might be
thought that because medical and nursing aims of restoring
him to health have failed, he is in more, rather than less, need
of comfort. Much work with the parents and family of a
handicapped child entails not solving a problem, but helping
them to live with it. This can be done by listening, and showing an understanding of the unhapppiness and frustration,
but perhaps most of all by sharing the problem. Mothers
in particular, who feel they are on their own contending with
an unusual baby, and trying to come to terms with their own
sometimes destructive feelings, and with the unspoken
comments of relatives and neighbours, carry a very heavy
burden.

The prognosis and possibilities for the baby have to be
dealt with from a medical angle. There may be surgical intervention which provides a long term hope of improvement. In

the short term, however, it removes the baby entirely from the mother's care, calls into question her competence as a mother, and disrupts the development of social behaviour between the two. Anything that can be done to maintain the contact between mother and baby may have long term consequences. With some help mothers can often provide much of the routine attention for their babies, even if they are seriously ill or recovering from an operation. There is the risk in hospital that nurses and midwives will take over the maternal role. One mother whose baby was in an incubator said to us, 'I am afraid the nurses will steal my baby'. She was expressing an anxiety often felt but seldom brought to the surface quite so clearly, that the intervention of a nurse between her and her baby might make her relationship with him less close.

Where there is no question of corrective or ameliorative surgery, the parents may face the prospect of caring of a baby with a poor prognosis. Unfortunately on this matter, as on most others with which we are concerned in this chapter, there is little in the way of systematic research which can help in framing a policy or advising parents. Most people would probably agree that caring for a dying child is a most distressing expereince. Babyhood and childhood are times for looking forward with hope. Dying is a time of grief and separation. The grief of bereavement is often anticipated by relatives and friends who are aware of the impending death. These incompatible emotions of hope and despair converge most painfully for anyone looking after a dying baby. The incongruity cannot be resolved. The excessive painfulness of the experience probably precludes the possibility of parents being able to express anything of it in words. Extremely painful experiences tend eventually to get repressed into the unconscious, where they are inaccessible to the normal processes of recollection. This almost certainly accounts for the fact that there is very little information available as to how parents cope with the conflicts and confusions aroused by a child with a short life expectation. An enquiry concerning visiting by parents to their babies in a special care unit, showed that they had to overcome very high levels of anxiety to visit. Even those parents, however, whose baby died, said they would have been very much against any restriction of visiting, and they did not regret any of the time they had spent with the child (Harper et al, 1976).

Parents of the abnormal or ill baby may have their instinctual responses of caring and protectiveness deflected by his appearance and prospects, but they may nevertheless be considerably motivated to do their best for their infant son or daughter. Any parent taking on such a task has a right to the relevant medical information which is available, and to have the assurance that support and help will be forthcoming when they need it.

The birth of a handicapped baby produces multiple insecurities. Even a mother who has had previous children, may have little to guide her as to how to physically handle her new baby. She is likely to wonder whether there are other associated handicapping conditions which she cannot see, or has not been told about. The birth may considerably upset her self-esteem, call into question her integrity as a wife, a mother, and a normal person. She may be unable to resolve a variety of questions in her own mind as to how the baby's siblings will be affected. Each mother will have her own characteristic way of responding, but it would be extraordinary if she did not show some unusual aspects of behaviour. The baby's father may also face a crisis over his self-esteem, integrity and manhood. A handicapped baby often arouses the whole family to self-examination. Difficult relationships between in-laws may explode into acrimonious genetic vilification with angry disappointed grandparents being anything but helpful. Anxiety and doubt may manifest themselves by ceaseless asking of questions. They may be straightforward requests for factual information, or used as a method of engaging someone's attention. If a question is repeatedly asked, despite an answer having been given, it may mean that the information is so totally unacceptable that it cannot be incorporated into the mother's thought processes. Most doctors and nurses will have had the experience of a patient, or patient's relative, claiming they have never been given an important, but disagreeable piece of information despite proof to the contrary. This often means the information when it *was* given, was so totally unacceptable to them that it has been subconsciously rejected. Anxieties are sometimes very difficult to put into words. All but the most articulate may not be asking quite the question they want to ask. They may be simply putting in a plea that someone should spare time to listen. Constant demands may be not for answers, but for someone to listen to anger, grief, self-accusation, despair or the blaming of others which may include the hospital, the obstetrician, or the midwife. This may be a testing out period too, in which the mother will find out who has the resources to help her, by sharing her unhappiness and making themselves available to her.

In most cases it will be impossible for a clear prognosis to be given. The early months and years will be wait-and-see period, with alternating hopes and fears. When future development is uncertain there is every reason to suggest to the parents, that the more interesting and stimulating the child's life can be made the better hope he will have for maximising his potential abilities.

THE HANDICAP THAT IS NOT OBVIOUS AT BIRTH

There is another class of handicapped babies. There are the ones in which no problem is immediately obvious. Many mentally subnormal children have shown no signs at birth of their handicapped status. The infant with Down's syndrome may not look abnormal to his parents, although the condition is usually suspected by hospital staff. The question then arises as to when, how, and by whom, the parents should be told. Parents have sometimes been left in ignorance until the child was more than two years old; some have discovered by accident. Others have been told almost immediately after the birth. It is not unknown for parents to have been misinformed that their baby has Down's syndrome. The debate as to the best time to give information derives from two opposing views. One is that where the diagnosis is certain, that parents have a right to have the information as soon as is practicable. The other view is that a normal loving relationship between mother and baby will have a better chance of development, without the intrusion of such information, and that it will be easier for the mother to accept the baby with his problem, after some social behaviour is established between the two.

An enquiry made of the mothers of 71 children with Down's syndrome born in the years 1950–56 in Edinburgh, showed that there was more satisfaction about the timing of their being told when this was done early than when it was done late (Drillien & Wilkinson 1964). 81.3 per cent of mothers who were informed before the baby was 10 days old said they were satisfied with the timing as compared with 22.2 per cent of them who were told after two years. It must be remembered, however, that these are mothers who have kept their babies. We do not know what proportion of all women who were told early rejected their babies. This certainly happens from time to time, and the damaging effect of this on the child's development makes it a serious consideration. The parents who leave their baby in hospital to be cared for, may be parents who would be unable to deal with stressful information at any time. As we have discussed elsewhere however, the first few days after birth are particularly sensitive to interferences. In any case it might be thought advisable to have the benefit of a chromosome analysis, which takes about four days, before making a pronouncement. (A diagnosis *can* be made within 24 hours from bone marrow. It seems doubtful whether this will be widely used for the diagnosis of Down's syndrome).

Outward appearances can be misleading. In the Edinburgh study mentioned above, nearly half the mothers said they realised there was something seriously wrong with their baby, before they were told. Five claimed to have recognised the stigmata when they first saw him. Retrospective information of this sort has to be treated with caution. The human memory is extremely unreliable, and we all tend to recall things which make sense in the light of later events, and we also recall *facts* which put us in a favourable light. On both these grounds mothers may recall having realised their child was unusual, rather earlier than was the case. A prospective study, that is one which keeps account of events as they happen, is needed to check on this kind of material.

There are, of course, parents who either observe peculiarities in their baby, or notice that nursing and medical staff behave unusually to the infant or to them. If the mother has not been informed and asks questions, it will not create an attitude of trust if she is fobbed off with some deceptive answer. Patients of every kind ought to be able to have complete trust in hospital staff, and to know that they are truthful. This is doubly important for parents of handicapped children, who will have to resort to professional advice and guidance more frequently than most. Doubts which are sown by their being misled on one occasion, may take a long time to dispel, as will the memory of a lack of sympathy or unkindness. There may be a period when, like the mother, the staff feel that the baby's appearance does arouse their suspicions, but perhaps it is better for them to insist that there is a period of ambiguity, until a chromosome analysis can be done. Parents are likely to be reluctant to acknowledge the fact that they have a handicapped baby. This can result in their not *taking-in* information they are given. It is important, therefore, that whoever tells them makes the condition of the baby quite clear and unequivocal. It is no kindness in the long run to allow ambiguity or false hope to creep in.

There is likely to be some agreed hospital policy on the matter of relaying information. When the diagnosis is confirmed with the parents, this should be given, together with some details of prognosis. At the same time, or very shortly afterwards, a careful explanation of the services that are available through the health and social services, and voluntary agencies can also be discussed. Perhaps most important is discussion about the positive aspects of the baby, and the important role the parents have to play in helping to make available to him the best facilities. Often enough parents of special or unusual children, have found their role as parents eroded by *experts*. They need the assurance that they can depend on getting help of the sort that will suit them and their family and that the *experts* will be available to help and advise as necessary.

The mentally retarded children who do relatively well, do so because their parents are caring, observant, responsive, and treat the child with respect and encouragement, setting their sights reasonably realistically. Some of the ground work for this, can be done during the puerperium, and the midwife can often teach some important lessons by her example. Some years ago it was confidently proclaimed by many doctors, that a child with Down's syndrome would never be able to learn to read or write. Many devoted teachers of the mentally handicapped have demonstrated the falsity of this assumption. The diary of Nigel Hunt published in 1967 is written by a young man with Down's syndrome who had been lovingly tutored by his mother.

TELLING THE PARENTS

Conveying bad news in never a pleasant task, and most of us avoid it when we can. Such information is probably better given initially by someone known to the parents, so that important features of their social circumstances are taken into account. A midwife who has looked after a woman during the antenatal period, and labour, and has made a good relationship with her, may be an appropriate person to introduce the parents to the fact that the baby has some abnormality which will affect his development. Some preliminary discussion of this sort, may help the parents to derive more benefit from their interview with the paediatrician, who will go into more detail and also be able to deal with long term prospects, and to give parents some idea of what lies ahead, as well as the services which are available. The social worker is an important member of the team, who will have more detailed information about the family, and is particularly skilled in dealing with the emotional difficulties arising.

The report of a working party of the National Association of Mental Health on 'The Birth of an Abnormal Child: Telling the Parents' (*Lancet* 1971) drew attention to the fact that some experienced workers advocate telling the father first. In the immediate post natal period, a father may be more stable than his wife and may appreciate the opportunity to be the first to talk with her about their baby. The report emphasises that on no account should he be used to transfer information which must come direct from a well informed member of the staff – normally the paediatrician.

The father however, is often bewildered and overwhelmed and making him party to such unwelcome information may be a great burden to him. As it is to be hoped that both parents will help and encourage the child, and each other, there seems much to be said for telling them both at the same time.

Abnormalities of the eyes and ears may not be apparent in the first two weeks of life. If defects are discovered by hospital staff, some debate may arise as to whether there is an immediate need to inform the parents. A similar question arises in conditions which may improve spontaneously, such as Erb's palsy. On the one hand it may be thought a disservice to the parents to give them cause for worry, when they are first embarking on settling down with their new baby – a task which comes smoothly to only a lucky few – and things may improve. On the other hand even minor sensory defects do effectively reduce the range and quality of stimulation to which a child can respond. This may affect his speed and pattern of development. Where parents are aware of a deficiency, they might also be able to compensate for it. For example if a baby is blind, or has poor vision, he needs to get more information about his surroundings by hearing and touch, and to develop these two modalities effectively. Were parents informed they could be helped to provide a richer and more varied range of experiences than might otherwise occur.

For a mother who has some difficulty in handling her new born baby, and gets readily upset, it may be better not to give her further cause for agitation. Generally, however, people manage situations better when they are informed than when they are not. If information about any adverse condition is given, it should be associated with possible corrective or ameliorative action which parents can take, and some outline of the prospects for the future.

Every newborn infant has a unique arrangement of innumerable traits and qualities. The baby who is described as handicapped lacks some feature, or characteristic, which is highly valued in our society. How far other features and characteristics can be developed in compensation, and how far he can be accepted as a valued human being, will depend on the environment in which he is reared. Whether he learns to think of himself as a whole person with an abnormality, or as an abnormal, second rate personality will depend on a variety of factors. For example, the way his parents and others accept him, the provision that is made available to help him develop his own special skills and abilities, and the social values that are daily and hourly communicated directly and inadvertently in casual conversations, in newspapers and television around him, all have an effect. By appreciating some of the problems the parents may face, the midwife can play an important part in giving information, sharing discussion and helping with appropriate emotional support.

REFERENCES

British Film Institute: (BFI) Experimental Production Board 1960 by Heather Sutton. Available from Concord Films, Ipswich.

Clifford, B. & Bull, R. (1976) *The Psychology of Personal Identification*. London: Routledge.

Drillien, C. M. & Wilkinson, E. M. (1964) Mongolism – When should parents be told? *British Medical Journal*, 22 pp 1306–7.

Harper, Rita, Sia, C., Sokal, S., Sokal, M. (1976) Journal of Paediatrics, 89 (3) pp 441–445.

Hewett, S. (1970) *The Family & the Handicapped Child*. London: Allen & Unwin.

Hunt, N. (1967) *The World of Nigel Hunt*. Chichester: Darwen Finlayson.

Kennell, J. H. Jerauld, R., Wolfe, H., Chesler, D., Kreger, N. C., McAlpine, W., Steffa, M. & Klaus, M. (1974) *Developmental Medicine & Child Neurology*, 16 pp 172–179.

Lansdown, R. & Polok, L. (1975) A Study of the Psychological Effects of Facial Deformity in Children. *Child Care, Health & Development*. 1 pp 85–91.

National Association of Mental Health (1971) The Birth of an Abnormal Child: Telling the Parents. *Lancet*, 2 pp 1075–1077.

Stillbirth

Occasionally a baby is stillborn. This poses a considerable number of problems as death for our society is rather as sex was for the Victorians; rarely talked of, surrounded with anxieties and embarrassment taking place secretly behind screens and curtains. Bereavement in these circumstances can rarely find suitable expression because it too, is a source of embarrassment. The rituals associated with the disposal of the dead body serve a number of important functions. A funeral which friends, relatives and neighbours attend, publicly affirms the altered status of the bereaved. A woman who has lost her baby is no longer a mother. It also affords the bereaved some formal outward sign of support. Attending a funeral in some parts of rural Britain is still regarded as a sign of respect for the bereaved family which it would be churlish to withhold. Another custom, now rarely practised, is to invite friends to look at the body in the coffin; the undertaker would leave the lid of the coffin unfastened until it reached the church, in case any mourners wanted to see the corpse. There are no doubt, some fairly material and practical explanations for this practice (for assurance that bodies had not been snatched or exchanged) but it also serves to enable members of the community to acknowledge their involvement and concern. At a psycho-social level such intimate

191

arrangements facilitated an easier communication about death, and a relative freedom from embarrassment.

PRACTICAL GUIDANCE

The Third Report of the Maternity Services Advisory Committee (HMSO 1985) includes a chapter on Stillbirths and Neonatal Deaths with some clear recommendations about support for parents, training for staff and counselling services for both. The practical guidance is to be welcomed, but above all, 'Parents should be given as much information as possible on the cause of their baby's death, be encouraged to discuss it and advised of any implication for the future.

GRIEVING

Much consideration has been given in the last few years to the management of a stillbirth. The problem of unresolved grief had been voiced by many parents who had been given no chance to see or touch their dead baby. This opportunity is now usually offered. Some mothers have found comfort in holding their dead baby in their arms, to acknowledge his brief existence in the spontaneous way that is quite appropriate with the newly born. A stillborn baby, although dead, has for months before, been a living being, of whom the mother has been aware. He has been growing, moving, been the focus for plans and hopes: his dying may seem the more desperate if the mother is denied the opportunity to touch or see the body, which has for so long been part of herself. It is not suggested that all mothers should see or hold their dead baby, but some have certainly regretted not having been allowed to do so. A short article by a midwife poignantly expressed this desire even though she realised her baby was macerated. Her midwife considered it inadvisable, but five months later the author was obviously still wishing she had seen the baby.

People who have not been present at the death of a relative or close friend have sometimes expressed a similar regret. There is a sense of incompleteness which makes mourning a more difficult process. In these cases of intra-uterine death the mother usually notices the absence of movements and realises that her labour will not produce a live baby. The immediate shock of death has often already passed. The unexpected stillbirth when the baby dies during labour or delivery, is a very different matter for both the parents and the staff. The quietness is bizarre. The midwife and obstetrician may have a sudden sense of failure of their professional abilities. The normal happy sequence of behaviour which follows delivery is totally disrupted; the usual words of encouragement, pleasure and admiration of the new baby dry up. The feelings of the staff may be in such disarray that they retreat into functional efficiency which can add to the anguish for the mother. It is a common experience for those associated with death to feel some guilt – was everything done as it should have been? – could things have been otherwise? The mother, bereft and stunned can be totally isolated with no longed-for baby, no words with which to communicate, and no one who can listen, or sit quietly with her. The deepest grief by being unspeakable may continue its corrosive work for years.

Some women, despite the fact that they have subsequently reared healthy children, continue to feel and grieve the loss of a stillbirth. When the subject is mentioned anger and distress are often still felt. One woman, known to us, said that she could hardly bear to think about it twenty years afterwards, and blushing deeply, apologised for having spoken of the event. Another attributed the breakup of her marriage to the fact that neither she nor her husband could deal with nor communicate their profound grief over their loss, possibly due to fear of deepening the wound to their partner even more.

How then can this situation be alleviated? Seeing or holding the baby, already mentioned, is helpful for some parents. For others, giving him or her a name serves the purpose of marking his brief life with some significance. Asking 'What is his name?' would perhaps help the mother to focus her anguish on a real person. Some mothers have been told to forget all about it and go home and start another baby as soon as possible. The implication seems to be that one baby is much the same as any other and the loss can be made good fairly quickly. For some mothers this may be the case although most women seem to recall in considerable detail, not the sameness of events associated with their children, but the differences. The marriage relationship develops and changes, and how the couple feel about each other is likely to be an important factor in their attitude to a new conception. Pregnancies are different too. Events that take place during the nine months contribute to the parents' ideas about the child. Bitter and unresolved grief is hardly a basis to be recommended for embarking on another pregnancy. Pregnancy is a time for looking forward and planning a new life, with which mourning for the stillborn must accord ill. The refusal to recognise the dead baby as having any personal significance for the mother may mean that she has to contend with free floating grief which she cannot locate in a person or a place. Depression is by no means uncommon in normal postnatal women, and in those who are at home for long periods (Gavron 1966, Lovegrove 1976). To be caught in addition, in a conspiracy to deny the importance of the pregnancy, the birth and death of a child, is highly likely to increase the risk of depression.

PLACE OF BURIAL

Traditionally the burial place has been of great significance. The tomb has been the object of pilgrimage, or of regular attention of some kind – placing of flowers or a wreath. Mothers do not always know the means by which their stillborn babies are disposed of, let alone know where their remains are to be found. 'We felt he had been buried like so much rubbish, with no acknowledgement of his much wanted, brief existence', wrote one mother (Jolly 1975). The practice of interring 'up to 299 bodies' of stillborn babies in a mass grave has apparently been done with the assumption 'that parents would never wish to visit their graves' (Times 1981). This is patently not the case. For some parents locating and tending the grave serves an important function.

What is clear is that problems associated with bereavement are often not effectively resolved in society as a whole, nor by health professionals (Parkes 1972). Stillbirth is a special case in which emotions associated with both birth and death become intertwined. The mother's body is hormonally prepared for a new life, the breasts fill for an infant who no longer lives. From the comments gleaned from a few mothers and from our own limited experience, this seems to be an area of personal relationships where much more needs to be known. How does the grief reaction differ from that for a person who has been well known? Further informaton concerning the long and short term effects of a stillbirth on parents, their grief reactions and their mourning processes, as well as the sort of help that is effective, is much needed. Little purpose seems to be served by imposing a taboo on seeing or speaking about the baby.

As this *death taboo* is a very general one in contemporary society it is often difficult for individuals to overcome. This applies as much to health professionals as to the general public. An event which is of great significance to an individual, but is nevertheless forbidden expression does not disappear. It is likely to remain the longer. It is the lot of many of the bereft to become social pariahs. The reason is that few of us know how to talk with them. We fear allowing them to talk as this may expose not only *their* unseemly feelings, but our own as well. To help a mother who has just borne a stillbirth a midwife needs, as well as an empathetic response to the mother, considerable self-understanding. This may come with experience of living, but can certainly be helped through discussion in suitably arranged group conditions. These can give some opportunity for members to reflect on their own intense feelings, some of which may be subject to strongly conditioned reticence.

A midwife who feels compelled to mask her own feelings by efficient busy-ness, is unlikely to be able to offer a mother much understanding if she should ask to hold her dead baby, or rail against the hospital and its staff, or lie mute in bed for her short stay in hospital. Holding the baby immediately after delivery is more practical than later on, when the little body is stiff and cold and has often been the subject of a post mortem examination. Preparing it then for viewing or holding, is a daunting task for anyone. Women who have had a stillbirth are usually discharged quickly from hospital. The presence of more fortunate women may, by providing contrast, exaggerate their grief, although it is likely that the core of the problem is the one already mentioned, namely the inhibitions and social embarrassments surrounding death and the bereaved. Undoubtedly every woman has her own way of contending with the disappointment and misery of still-birth. Adversities which do not overwhelm can initiate personal growth, but if they are too great they can have a damaging effect on a person's functioning which may be protracted or even permanent. In the last twenty or so years there has been a great interest in the psychological aspects of dying, and bereavement, and a few pioneers like Dame Cecily Saunders have helped, not only to change provision for care, but have considerably altered public and professional attitudes. A similar change of attitude to, and treatment of, parents who have had stillbirths is now apparent.

STILLBIRTH AND NEONATAL DEATH SOCIETY

The Stillbirth and Neonatal Death Society (SANDS) was estab-lished in 1978, in response to pleas for help from parents who had experienced stillbirths and other perinatal and neonatal deaths. The aims of the Society are:

(i) To establish a national network of parents who are willing to help others who have been similarly bereaved;

(ii) To enable doctors, midwives and other professionals to be more aware of the feelings and needs of parents at the time of their bereavement;

(iii) To encourage research into the causes of perinatal death and effects on the family;

(iv) To make the public more aware of the needs and long-term effects of such deaths on the family.

The address of the Society can be found on page 210. An information pack for professionals is available from SANDS called 'Stillbirth and Neonatal Death–what happens next?' The Health Education Council in conjunction with SANDS and the National Association for Mental Health have produced an eleven page leaflet (1985) called 'The loss of your baby at birth or shortly after'. This includes some guidance on practical arrangements that have to be made for registering the death and arranging the funeral. In an attempt to reduce the stress to parents and staff when a baby dies some Health Authorities have devised a specific policy for action. Instructions may be set down as to who is responsible for informing the parents, arrangements to be made for the delivery and postpartum care of the mother; arrangements to be made with the Registrar of Births & Deaths; for the funeral, and with the general practioner. 'Familiarity with these practical issues facilitates an entrée to bereavement counselling for the parents' it is claimed (Forrest et al 1981) As many newly bereaved parents cannot respond positively to offers of counselling and support this is an important observation. Parkes (1980) in reviewing the efficacy of bereavement counselling concluded that it can reduce the psychiatric and psychosomatic disorders that result from bereavement.

REFERENCES

Forrest, G. C., Claridge, R. S. & Baum, J. D. (1981) *British Medical Journal*, **282** pp 31–32.
Gavron, H. (1966) *The captive wife*. London: Penguin. Health Education Council (1985) *The Loss of Your Baby*.
Jolly, H. (1975) The heartache of facing the facts of the stillborn baby. *The Times*, 3 December.
Lovegrove, S. (1976) *Stuck at Home*. London:BBC Publications.
Parkes, C. M. (1972) *Bereavement: Studies of Grief in Adult Life*. London: Tavistock Publications.
Parkes, C. M. (1980) Bereavement counselling: does it work? (British Medical Journal, **281** pp 3–6.

13

Going home

Patients are usually delighted to go home. After the grati-
tudes, the thanks, the words of advice the most important
thing is to get home to independence, to be on one's own
territory and to work things out. An additional member of a
family alters its structure (that is the way members relate to
each other). A first baby necessitates quite considerable
adaptation in the relationship between husband and wife.
Their concerns and conversations will change and their attention will be divided between the baby and their partner. This
applies particularly to the mother who may find that the
demands the baby makes necessarily reduce the time she can
spend with her husband.

JEALOUSY OF THE NEW BABY

The second baby in turn alters a mother's relationship with
both her husband and the first child. Jealousy is the likely
outcome if attention which a person believes should rightly
be theirs is diverted elsewhere. It is an emotion, by no means
unheard of, in fathers of first babies and is almost universal
in first children if the second born arrives at a critical stage
of his development. Sewell (1930) found that jealousy in the

first sibling is likely when the second baby is born when he is between 18 and 42 months. This is exactly the time when most families have their second baby. From a physiological and family planning point of view the spacing of two to three years has much to recommend it. Parents can perhaps be encouraged, before the new baby goes home, to pay special attention to the older child, or children, and to incorporate all members of the family in caring for the new baby (Fig. 13.1). The problem is specially acute when the second birth is a multiple one. The two and a half year old first born daughter of a family known to us was transformed from a reasonable and happy child to a murderous little virago when her twin siblings came home. Her mother had had to be in hospital for longer than usual. From the child's point of view she had been abandoned by her mother, who, when she eventually returned, devotedly attended to two interlopers. The emotional power generated by such an experience may remain a permanent feature, although it usually takes a more socially acceptable direction later in life. It is a circumstance which is difficult to cure, but which much might be done to prevent, by maintaining contact between mother and older child, keeping her informed, getting her to share the care of the babies, but otherwise minimising contact with them in her presence.

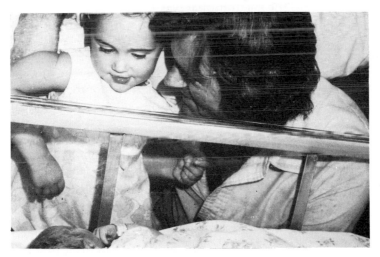

Figure 13.1 Older child being encouraged to join in.

Husbands who feel jealous can express their feelings and are aware of the source of their moodiness. Small children however cannot say what it is that angers them and they may become hostile and difficult to get on with. Not only are young children likely to be jealous of the new baby, but they can react badly to the mother's absence. If the mother has been in hospital for a week or ten days, and they were inadequately prepared for her departure, they may feel that she has abandoned them. When she returns, instead of being greeted by a welcoming little son or daughter, she may be given a very cold shoulder.

REARRANGEMENT OF RELATIONSHIPS

Young children separated from their mother can go through the stages of protest withdrawal and despair. The separation can create in them a feeling of insecurity, which may show itself in clinging and demanding behaviour. The mother who goes home to a toddler, may find that she has to contend with a new baby and a child who has regressed in his social behaviour. The mother may find that she is put out, too, over a number of small things. She may find that the family have got on remarkably well without her. Instead of being welcomed into the vacuum that was left by her departure, she finds that people are tardy in making room for her. 'We've done it this way for the past ten days' her husband or her mother may say, as she settles into an accustomed task . . . or 'I've altered the furniture in the living room while you were away; you have been wanting it done for months.' She may be pleased the job is done, but regretful that it could be done without her.

A mother can also feel very possessive about her baby and resent the time her husband spends with him. Being a member of a family has problems as well as pleasures. The rearrangement of relationships that has to occur with a new member joining the family, may take a little while to sort out and will need patience. The number of potential relationships in a group multiplies rapidly as the number of members increases. A three person group can relate to each other like this:

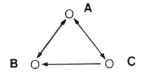

But A may also relate to B & C who act in unison on some matter.

Let us add two more people:-

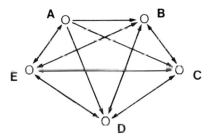

Each member can relate to every other individual. A however may sometimes have to deal with B C D & E combined, or B & C, and D & E and so on.

For those who like formulae here are two. The first one is the formula for calculating the number of single relationships and the second is more complex and gives in addition the possible ways members can group themselves and act in concert.

$$1. \quad X = \frac{n^2 - n}{2}$$

$$2. \quad X = \frac{3n - 2^{n+1} + 1}{2}$$

Where X = number of relationships
n = number of individuals

Table 13.1 shows the number of potential relationships there are in groups of different sizes.

Table 13.1

Number of members	Simple one to one relationships (Formula 1)	Complex relationships (Formula 2)
2	1	1
3	3	6
4	6	25
5	10	90
6	15	301
7	21	966

You will see that in addition to problems of jealousy, role change, and allocation of territory, the addition of say a third child, increases the potential number of relationships from 25 to 90 (Hare 1962).

SPECIAL FEATURES OF FIRST BORN CHILDREN

There is considerable evidence that many first born children develop in rather different ways from subsequent children (Altus 1966, Sampson 1962, Bartlett and Smith 1966). First born children tend to be more independent and to be higher achievers. One of the explanations put forward for this is that the first born is the only child in a family who has his parents to himself for a period, and then has to share them. No matter how understanding the parents, or how much they may compensate to the first born, the inescapable fact is that when the second baby arrives he experiences the loss of the undivided attention of his mother and father. One view about the first born, is that he can never again take the love of his parents for granted, but has to win their affection. The longing to be reinstated motivates the child to show how worthy he is of parental affection. This may become a permanent character trait, impelling him to achieve highly throughout life. First and only children are often expected to be more responsible than later born children in the family.

Another important factor with the first born is that it is generally the first experience for the parents with *any* baby. They therefore do a lot of learning, and perhaps make a lot of mistakes with the first one. Most parents would agree that they are more anxious with their first born. The mother may look at her sleeping baby every twenty or thirty minutes to assure herself that he is still breathing. When the second one arrives she is so much more confident and relaxed that she will not peer anxiously at him so frequently! Most parents remember a lot about their first baby – when he first sat up, spoke, walked, as well as innumerable amusing stories about his early adventures. With each successive member of the family, the details of the child's birth and development may be less and less precisely recalled.

In addition there is a higher rate of abnormality during the pregnancy, labour and delivery with first babies. This may mean that the first borns are in general rather more difficult children to manage.

EFFECTS ON NEW MOTHERS OF BEING AT HOME

Urban industrialised societies have predominantly a nuclear family structure. That is mother, father and children form an independent unit. The extended family consisting not only of mother, father and children, but grandparents, uncles and aunts, which characterises some of the less advanced societies, has a number of advantages for the new mother which is lacking in Britain. Children in extended families can experience multiple-mothering which releases the mother from the entire twenty-four hour a day responsibility for the care of her young. There is now appreciable evidence that many mothers of pre-school children are unable to enjoy the company of their youngsters on account of being depressed, socially isolated and miserable. Epidemiological studies, looking at women in the community, show how very common is depression in mothers of children aged under five and how widespead its effect can be on family life and on children's development and health (Wolkind 1981). From an active economic and social life, many have to adapt to financial dependence and severe social limitations. Despite sentimental attitudes, the mother role is not highly valued in this society, which takes its measure from more specifically task directed roles. Many people, especially men, when asked who they are describe themselves in terms of a task: 'I am a bus driver', 'I am a teacher' but full-time mothers will often say 'I am only a mum'. 'I am *only* . . .' is a denigrating self assessment.

Mothers who are more positive about their role (as they often are if they have a challenge to deal with e.g. a handicapped child) occasionally find themselves compelled to assert their position vis a vis the specialist teacher, pediatrician, health visitor, and social worker. There is no specific training for motherhood as there is for bus driving and teaching. In the specialisation which occurs with advance in society, parenting has been left out, and is done well or ill on the basis of casual labour. A few voices have been raised in a plea for parentcraft classes for both boys and girls from school days onward. So far however such classes are rather casual and *ad hoc*.

We have a society of one family units, where work is quite separate from the home, in which motherhood is not a highly regarded task. In some urban areas the position for mothers is made worse by the architectural lunacy of having people live on top of one another instead of side by side. We talk to people whom we meet face to face, not people who live *above* or *below* us. In consequence a very common complaint by the mothers of young children, is that they are lonely, bored, depressed, stuck-at-home and unfulfilled. Not the ideal atmosphere for a baby to develop into a joyful, exploring, curious, bright and interested child.

HELPING YOUNG MOTHERS TO AVOID ISOLATION

A midwife cannot alter our nuclear family structure nor the architecture of the towns. There is much that mothers can do in the way of self help and the midwife may be in a good position to make relevant suggestions. Young mothers groups are sometimes based on the local health visitors' clinic. They may meet to discuss common problems, to exchange children's clothes and equipment, and deal with a variety of practical and social matters. A few mothers can combine to form a babysitting group so that each member can leave her baby for a couple of hours with someone who is known, and who will become a firm acquaintance of the child as well. In some areas there are classes with a crèche attached organized by a voluntary group, or the Local Authority. Classes on a wide range of topics can often be arranged in response to a specific request by a local group. The absence of stimulation, both social and intellectual, can be sorely felt. Boredom and isolation have their effects, not only by making people *feel* dreary; they have a disabling effect on thinking, on psycho-motor skills, on the ability to plan and think ahead and indeed affect the whole personality. A guiding word from the midwife which will encourage the new mother to think what active steps she can take to combat these risks may have permanent value.

The mother who comes from a cohesive family is specially fortunate. She can look forward to sharing the experience of caring for the baby with her husband and may also have help from her mother who can build up her confidence. The problem of the grandmother usurping the mother's role is a well-known one. This may be a special risk if grandmother has recently retired from a job, or lost her husband, or for some other reason is making a new role for herself.

THE UNSUPPORTED MOTHER

Some others will be going home without the help and support of a husband. We have discussed in Chapter 4 important differences between being unmarried and unsupported. What matters to mother and baby is that they can return to a home where care and affection are shown. Some patients cannot look forward to such a welcome. A baby brought up without a permanent male figure in the house may be at a long-term disadvantage. His mother, however, needs some supportive person as soon as she leaves hospital. Looking after a young baby is not an easy job for the inexperienced and untutored. In addition the unsupported mother is likely to have worries about practical matters that a more fortunate woman is spared. Despite more liberal attitudes, having a baby without an identifiable male support is a social disadvantage. Probably the only exception to this is the woman whose husband has died during the pregnancy. A woman on her own, needs to be exceptionally capable to make provision for her children in a way that would compare with the two-parent family.

The single mother may be resentful, guilty or bereft at being on her own. She may be afflicted with many doubts about her relationships and her competence. However satisfactorily she comes to terms with events, caring for a young child single handed is a further strain. She should be referred to the social worker before she goes home, so that every form of support available can be offered.

MOTHER WITH A HANDICAPPED BABY

The mother with the handicapped child may have to go home before her baby is fit enough to be discharged from hospital. This in itself is a problem. Is she a mother or not? One of the requirements of the mother role is that the baby should be cared for. If she is not competent to care for him, she forefeits the role. The precariousness of the infant's status affects hers, and for the time until her baby can come home she is likely to be in a state of limbo. Much of the time in hospital will have been devoted to considering the prospects for the baby and making plans for the future. The parents, in their relationships with staff, may have begun to adjust to the idea of having a child with a handicap. Once at home the whole process has to be gone through again with neighbours and friends. If the handicap is perceived as a minor one an attitude of guarded optimism and encouragement for the new mother may prevail. Many parents have found that the embarrassment of a major handicapping condition serves only to turn them in upon themselves. Neighbours do not speak because they do not know what to say. Neither rejoicing nor commiseration seem appropriate. The parents' response of not initiating contact is predictable, and they run the serious risk of becoming more and more socially isolated. This may have a souring effect on them, and hinder the child's prospects of development.

With the prevailing policy of care in the community for the mentally ill and handicapped there is, perhaps, greater familiarisation of the population generally with handicapped people. The degree of successful integration which can in practice be effected is likely to colour attitudes to handicapping conditions. If the handicapped can reasonably take their place in the community rather than being 'put away', attitudes may be more accepting and relaxed.

The midwife may be able to discuss these problems with the mother before she goes home. The prospects for the individual child can never be predicted with absolute accuracy. While it would be irresponsible and unkind to encourage false optimism, it is quite realistic to press the view that whatever the child's handicap his chances of developing his potential can best be helped by the provision of social and mental stimulation by affectionate parents. In practical terms this means taking him to the shops, and to visit friends, talking and playing with him, providing him with play things, and later on playmates. A mother of a child with a handicap should be encouraged to view her baby as the repository of unknown potential which she has the important function of helping him to discover. The ratio of disappointment and frustration to joy and achievement, may be different from that with a normal child. The maintenace of the parents' own social lives is of great importance too, if they are to avoid an accumulation of the stresses imposed by a handicap in the family.

Some mothers are so distressed at the prospect of living with a handicapped child that they abandon him to the hospital from whence he must sooner or later be transferred to the care of the Local Authority. It is undoubtedly right that the community generally should take a share in the disproportionate demands made by a child with a serious disability. In community support can be effectively channelled through the parents, the benefits to the child can be inestimable. The fact that some parents do abandon their children, is a measure of the failure, as the parents see it, of the community to make its supportive services clearly available.

The health visitor has a duty to visit parents of pre-school children after they leave the care of the midwife. It is to the health visitor that the parents may turn for help and advice in the early days at home. Before leaving hospital the mother is given an appointment for a postnatal check. In addition to these universally available services, we give in the Appendix some addresses of organisations which may be of help to parents for themselves, and in connection with special problems they may have with their babies (see p. 209–211).

The physical, social and emotional conditions in which children are conceived, carried, born, fed and nurtured contribute to the moulding of their personalities, and affect the families into which they are born. Midwives have a distinctive and irreplaceable contribution to make to this vital developmental stage. They have long been recognised as competent to deal with the physical aspects of normal pregnancy, labour and puerperium, and many practising midwives will from their experience, have developed intuitive insights beyond much of what we have written. We hope, however, that this book may help to clarify the basis of their understanding. We hope, too, that future midwives and parents may have sufficient confidence in themselves to make their appropriate contribution to the childbearing process. It is an event of critical importance to the life of the child, to the next generation and to the society of the future.

REFERENCES

Altus, W. D. (1966) Birth order and its sequelae. *Science*, **151** 44–49.
Bartlett, E. W. & Smith, C. P. (1966) Child rearing practices, birth order and the development of achievement related motives. *Psychological Reports*, **18** 1207–1216.
Hare, A. Paul. (1962) *Handbook of Small Group Research*. London: Collier MacMillan Ltd.
Sampson, E. E. (1962) Birth order, need achievement and conformity.
    Journal of Abnormal and Social Psychology, **64** 155–159.Sewell, M. (1930)
Sewell, M. (1930) Some causes of jealousy in young children. *Study of Social Work*, **1** 23–40.
Wolkind, S. (1981) Depression in mothers of young children. *Archives of Disease in Childood*, **56** pp 1–3.

Appendix

Where to look for help for parents and their young children

This list is very short. There are many organisations, both statutory and voluntary, set up to deal with specific and general needs. These few suggestions we hope will provide ideas as to where to begin.

General

Statutory services. The general practitioner and health visitor work within the Health Authority. Their addresses and telephone numbers can be found in the telephone book or from the local town hall.

The social worker is an employee of the Local Authority and can be contacted in the same way.

For single parents

'Gingerbread' , 35 Wellington Street, WC2, London. Telephone 01-240-0953.

National Council for One Parent Families , 255 Kentish Town Road, NW5 2LX. Telephone 01-267-1361. Gives advice on legal and financial matters, offering a counselling service and working for improvement in the services.

For the family with a handicapped child

An invaluable source of information will be found in *A handbook for Parents with a Handicapped Child* by J Stone and F Taylor, published by Arrow Books Ltd, 1977.

Association for Spina Bifida and Hydrocephalus, 23 Upper Woburn Place, London WC1. Telephone 01-388-1352, and has 70 local associations.

Down's Children's Association, 4 Oxford Street, London, W1. Telephone 01-580-0511

Invalid Children's Aid Association, 126 Buckingham Palace Road, London, SW1 9SB. Telephone 01-730-9891

Spastics Society, 12 Park Crescent, London, W1N 4EQ. Telephone 01-636-5020.

For the family who have lost a baby at birth or later

Stillbirth and Neonatal Death Society (SANDS) Argyle House, Euston Road, NW1, London. Telephone 01-833-2851.

For the family who had a cot death

Foundation for the Study of Infant Deaths, 5th Floor, 4 Grosvenor Place, London SW1X 7HD. Telephone 01-235-1721 or 01-245-9421.

For the family with a gifted child

National Association for Gifted Children, 1, South Audley, London W1 Telephone 01-499-1188.

For the parents

Workers Educational Association, (WEA), 9, Upper Berkeley Street, London W1 H8B. Telephone 01-402-5608. The WEA have local branches in most parts of the country. Morning or afternoon classes, with crêche facilities are run where there is a local demand, although most of the educational work is done in evening classes.

National Housewives Register, c/o Josephone Jaffray, Holmshaw, Moffat, Dumfries, DE10 95Q. Telephone Beattock

422. For women who can develop activities including paid work, from their own homes.

For the pregnant woman

Association for Improvements in the Maternity Service, 21 Iver Lane, Iver, Bucks. Telephone Iver 652781.

National Childbirth Trust, 9, Queensborough Terrace, London W2. Telephone 01-221-3833. An educational charity providing antenatal preparation for parents, help with breast feeding, as well as seminars and study days.

Foundation for Education and Research in Childbearing, 27, Walpole Street, London, SW3. Telephone 01-730-0710. Disseminated information on all aspects of childbearing.

National Birthday Trust, 57, Lower Belgrave Street, London, SW1. Telephone 01-730-5607. Initiates and supports research into aspects affecting maternal welfare.

Index